YOU'RE SHARP ENOUGH
TO BE YOUR OWN SURGEON:

The Body Contouring Programme™

KEITH D. CLARK, MA, DCH

Transpersonal
☼Publishing

ISBN 1-929661-16-9

First Printing, August 1993
2nd Printing, June, 2005
Cover Illustration by Pau Publications, LTD.

For additional retail copies of this book, go to:

www.holistictree.com

For additional wholesale quantities of this book or other related
books, tapes, and CDs, contact the publisher through the worldwide
web:
www.TranspersonalPublishing.com

Transpersonal
:Ö: Publishing
div. AHU, LLC
PO Box 249
Goshen, VA 24439

Manufactured in the United States of America
10 9 8 7 6 5 4 3 2 1

YOU'RE SHARP ENOUGH
TO BE YOUR OWN SURGEON:
The Body Contouring Programme™

Table of Contents

A Ohe Pau Ko Ike I Kou Halau

"Think not that all wisdom is in your school"

- Ancient Hawai'ian Saying

March 26, 1993

Somewhere in Hakalau. Hakalau is a Hawai`ian word for a heightened state of defocused attention, which I also use to describe a particular type of trance, as well as a small community on the east side of the big island of Hawai`i, in North Hilo District. Somewhere in Hakalau, it is here that much of the teaching, much of the thought, and much of the actual work has been done. It's time to put these thoughts and information into print. Time to put the words down. This is where the knowledge begins, here in Hakalau.

Robert & Jeanne

Mahalo

Acknowledgments

There have been many individuals who have been directly and/or indirectly responsible for the effectiveness of the techniques contained within this book. I would first like to begin by thanking Professor Barbara Bullard at Orange Coast College for first exposing me to visualization in 1974. She has remained an exquisite friend, colleague and mentor over the years. Dr. A. M. Krasner at the American Institute of Hypnotherapy (AIH) for the opportunity to develop myself and this program with the assistance of AIH. Dr. Tad James as a Master Trainer of Neuro Linguistic Programming (NLP), the development of Time Line Therapy™ and his continuing friendship and encouragement over the years. Jill Dianne for her unique view of the world, which continually allowed me to clarify and identify the techniques that I utilize in order that they may be more easily taught and understood. Robert Smith for the light hearted encouragement and infinite insights into possibilities. Uncle George Naope for continued Aloha. To all of the unnamed individuals whom I have seen as clients and engaged in conversation over the years to gain insights into being human being.

Preface

by Dr. Tad James

Dr. Clark's *Body Contouring Programme*™ is a landmark in the field of Hypnosis and psychology. He has done an excellent job in capturing the essence of the program. This book clearly explains the steps and allows the reader to discover the scope of the program.

For years, as I have done Time Line Therapy™ with clients, I have been interested in how our self-image leads to our physical condition. In working with thousands of clients over the years, I began to notice that one could predict something about their present problem, just by looking at them. In addition, I would notice that once a client told me their problem that I could see its reflection in their external physical appearance. Then as we completed our time together, I noticed that the client's appearance would change as if by magic. I know that when I told them "You look different," often it was beyond the scope of their beliefs. Unless they also felt different inside, they were not as

Programme^{TM} seems to produce results on the outside and on the inside.

The entire *Body Contouring Programme*^{TM} is explained here, and is laid out in a way that makes it easy to get started right away. Using Time Line Therapy^{TM} we discover how to clean up issues in our past such as fear, uncertainty, confusion, trauma, unworthiness, limiting decisions, resentment. The contribution of competition and role models to body image is also examined. Using proven methods of Hypnosis, we learn how to use our imagination to restructure our body. Through the field of Neuro Linguistic Programming we find that our innermost thoughts can actually support us in becoming who we want.

The book is an easy to use "How to" program with suggestions about what to do and when to do it.

All in all the book is easy for the average reader to use and a contribution to the field -- a rare contribution, and well worth reading. If you have any interest in the body-mind connection for physical change, this is the book. This book is a "must have" for anyone interested in self-image! Enjoy it.

-- Tad James, M.S., Ph.D., is an author, lecturer, and personal development consultant. He is the author of *Time Line Therapy and the Basis of Personality*, and *The Secret of Creating Your Future*.

Introduction

We are complex in the simplicity of our human-ness, and our being-ness. This body of work draws upon an interconnected network of concepts, none of which is more fundamental than another. As we present here the progression of the theory, the interconnections in this network come more and more into focus.

This book has been written in response to the many doctors and therapists who have requested more information on the techniques we have found to be effective in assisting others to achieve changes in their physical shape. This is a technique we call *Body Contouring*™. The process itself is called *The Body Contouring Programme*™. The conceptual framework underlying this process perceives the human organism as a dynamic system involving interdependent physiological and psychological patterns.

During the 1940's Maxwell Maltz, M.D., F.I.C.S., published his book *New Faces--New Futures*, a collection of case histories where cosmetic surgery, particularly facial cosmetic surgery, had opened the door to a new life for many people. In that publication Maltz described the "amazing changes that often occurred in a person's personality" following cosmetic surgery. Maltz relates his amazement at the "dramatic and sudden changes in character and personality" which often resulted when a facial defect was corrected. Such amazement and his desire to understand more fully the phenomenon he witnessed led to research in the field he identified as "self-image psychology". From that research and inquiry he ultimately wrote and published *Psycho-Cybernetics* (1960). Maltz presented options for bettering your life, achieving peace of mind, giving yourself an emotional face lift, for turning failures into successes. He suggested the possibility that whether a person changed their external appearance with cosmetic surgery, or not, changing one's internal picture, could lead to feeling better about oneself and a better quality of life.

If altering the physical appearance through the utilization of cosmetic surgery could change an individual's personality, Maltz suggested that changing an individual's 'face of personality' or, self-image, could improve the quality of life. We suggest taking that premise to the next, natural step.

To paraphrase Deepak Chopra, M.D., author of *Ageless Body, Timeless Mind* (1993), quantum theorists tell us that rather than being composed of atoms, as was popular thought, 'solid' matter is made up of subatomic particles; particles of energy and information in a void of energy and information. The 'real' or tangible world in which we exist is formed by these particles of energy and information. The mind utilizes energy and information to create our feelings, ideas, instincts, desires and they are very real; they form the physical world in which we exist. Thoughts create war, the Berlin Wall, holes in the ozone layer and ballistic missiles. They also create harmony, laughter, love, a lack of aging and the body in which you live.

We suggest that change in an individual's self-concept - the internal picture or personal mental blueprint - in addition to improving self-esteem, can and does alter that individual's external, physical appearance.

The Body Contouring Programme^{TM} consists of a complete make-over, mentally, emotionally and physically. The techniques and processes involved in *The Body Contouring Programme*^{TM} are the eclectic result of twenty years of study, application and observation of the mental processes employed by individuals. Numerous philosophies, beliefs, and theories have been explored and synthesized into this effective technique.

Unlike other research, techniques and therapies targeted only at increasing the breast size of the client, *The Body Contouring Programme*^{TM} addresses all aspects of the individual mentally, emotionally and physically. *The Body Contouring Programme*^{TM} has proven effective in providing "spot reductions" in specific areas for the client. In addition, several other areas of desirable changes have occurred.

The Body Contouring Programme^{TM} is designed to work compatibly with the mental and emotional needs of the client as well as the physical. The majority of participants involved in *The Body Contouring Programme*^{TM} report a much improved quality of life, self-esteem and mental outlook. There has also been virtually unanimous consensus as to an increase in energy level as well as increased

increased sensuality and sensitivity. These internal changes were reported in addition to the outwardly noticeable physical changes.

As mentioned previously, this book has been written to satisfy the many requests from doctors and therapists interested in the physical, emotional and mental processes addressed by our program. **This book has not been written as a "how to" manual for self-transformation.** However, at the risk of sounding contradictory, the trained individual should be able to utilize the theory and techniques described within the text to experience comparable results with clients or for yourself.

As doctors, therapists and as individuals, we must realize that all change comes from within the individual. In authoring this work I am offering you, the readers, the opportunity to share in our successful theory and techniques. Upon gaining a full understanding of this material, you too should be able to assist yourself and others with the tools and insights necessary to assist in completing a successful *Body Contouring Programme*™.

Research exists from the early 1960's on the successful use of hypnosis with subjects desiring breast enlargement, and more recently, on the reduction of fat cells. Currently the practice of liposuction is widely accepted as the preferred surgical procedure employed to accomplish fat cell reduction. However, in contrast to surgical techniques, the use of hypnosis has been widely accepted for weight reduction for a number of years. Thousands of people every year experience successful results in weight reduction through the use of hypnosis. In addition, hypnosis has proven highly effective in behavior modification. More recent and advanced technologies such as Neuro

Linguistic Programming and Time Line Therapy™ are currently emerging as the preferred therapies for behavioral changes.

The Body Contouring Programme™ was developed to provide women an alternative to cosmetic surgery, breast implant surgery, liposuction, extreme diets and excessive exercise plans. Since its conception, it has evolved into a program which can accommodate any individual desiring physical change. The techniques included within *The Body Contouring Programme*™ have been utilized in hair restoration, behavioral modification, performance enhancement and symptom treatment. We invite you to utilize these techniques. As you experience your own success dare to go beyond what is currently known, further expanding this exciting and rewarding field.

The Body Contouring Programme™ combines elements of creative visualization, imagery, hypnosis, Neuro Linguistic Programming, Time Line Therapy™ and specific language patterns. We now offer you the opportunity to learn about this highly effective program. The combination of these advanced therapy techniques have never before been so effectively combined for use in the area of specific physical change. Furthermore, we invite you to seek out a *Body Contouring Programme*™ practitioner with which to work. You may even have the desire and qualifications to become a *Body Contouring Programme*™ practitioner yourself.

I

Mental and Physical States

Chapter One

Bodymind

It is important to have an understanding of the historical division between body and mind. Perhaps more appropriately put, rather than division, the lack of acceptance of anything other than observable matter having any influence or connection with our physical body. There has clearly been (and in many areas still is) a denial, particularly in Western culture, of anything having influence over an individual's body that is not of an organic nature. Any connection between the physical body and the mind was nonexistent. As a matter of fact, the concept of the mind existing at all is relatively new in Western culture. So at this initial point we shall first discuss some of the qualities of both the physical body and the mind. We will then proceed to discuss the interconnectedness of both the body and the mind. Indeed, a basic premise of this program is the concept that mind, body and spirit are interconnected.

Physiological Framework

The physical body that each of us possess (or possesses us) is made up of roughly 50 trillion cells. About 30 billion of these are nerve cells. Every day millions of cells throughout our bodies are being replaced. This takes place through the normal process of attrition and replacement. Indeed 98% of our body is replaced within one year. The remaining cells are replaced the following year. In fact, 10% of all cells in your body are replaced every 3 weeks, 25% of the cells are replaced every 5-6 weeks. The cells that make up our skin is totally new every thirty days. The cells that make up the soft muscle tissue of our internal organs is replaced in two to three months. The liver is replaced within six weeks, while the stomach lining takes as little as four days. Some cells, such as those closely involved in the process of digestion, are replaced as rapidly as every five minutes!

The understanding of how rapidly the body re-creates itself is quite encouraging. In his book *Quantum Healing* Dr. Deepak Chopra uses the analogy of the body as a river. Just as the river is constantly flowing, full of varying speeds of movement, so do the replacement of cells in our bodies. We are not merely stagnant physical beings that age and ultimately die. We are, in contrast, being ever renewed. Understanding this means realizing that next year you be an entirely different person than you are now. No matter what you do in the next twelve months, at least on a cellular level, you will be an entirely different person.

The process that the human body uses to deliver nutrients is *complexly simple*. Complex, in that we could not fully describe the entire process within this book. Simple, in its basic components. We ingest food, air, water and sunlight. Our internal organs and glands break-down, process, derive and create the nutrients that our bodies require. Our blood then transports the needed nutrients to the appropriate part of the body. Part of the transportation provided by the blood includes both "delivery and pick-up". In other words the blood delivers the nutrients as well as other components, while also removing the discarded components of the physical body. When the nutrients are delivered throughout the body they are used to nurture existing and create replacement cells as needed.

Knowing that the cells in our bodies are constantly changing gives us the option of replacing the old cells with stronger, healthier ones. An athlete in training pushes their body to new limits. Their body responds by replacing old cells with new ones better adapted to meet the demands being placed upon them. To further assist their body in creating these cellular changes an athlete will pay close attention to the quality and quantities of nutrients they consume. The more appropriate the fuel, the more easily and rapidly the desired changes can occur.

This theory is fairly easy for most people to accept. Why then would they not expect their body to adapt to sitting at a desk or on a sofa and consuming "junk" food? It certainly makes sense that if the body adapts to one type of stimulus that bit will surely adapt to another. In either case the body is responding to physical elements, food and exercise (or lack of it).

As we pointed out, our physical body is the compilation and incredibly exact construction and interaction of roughly 50 trillion cells. However, the actual complexity of cells is not yet fully understood. We do know that all cells in the body have components shared by every other cell in the body. This common denominator is DNA. The DNA code was discovered in the early 1950's by Watson and Crick. Its discovery has attempted to explain many of the qualities that cells possess. The presence of DNA is now widely accepted as being the primary building block and keeper of our genetic code.

Recently there has been new exception taken to this now widely held belief. Researchers such as Dr. Bruce Lipton present the view that DNA couldn't possibly contain all of the characteristics and responsibilities that are attributed to it. Lipton presents the view that the cell has an *intelligence* and responds to its environment, creating whatever is needed in order for the cell to evolve and survive. The cell is actually communicating to some extent in response to its environment.

The contemporary British physicist David Bohm theorized the notion of *unbroken wholeness*. This is based upon a belief that all of reality is held in place by an invisible field that knows what is happening everywhere simultaneously. He described this with the analogy of a hologram. In this hologram each part, in some sense, contains the whole. If any part of a hologram is illuminated, the entire image will be reconstructed. In Bohm's view the real world is structured according to the same general principles, with the whole enfolded in each of its parts. Within each cell, each atom, each subatomic particle, within each thought, whim or desire is the potential for creation and manifestation in our *real* world. This theory, while somewhat accepted, has yet to be proven.

Quantum theorists now tell us that where in the past it was generally held that matter was composed of atoms, we now see that atoms are composed of subatomic particles - which are fluctuations of energy and information in a void of energy and information.

To use the words of Sir Arthur Eddington, a British astronomer of the 19th century, "*the stuff of the world is mind-stuff.*" The essential stuff of the universe, including your body, is non-stuff, but it isn't ordinary non-stuff. It is thinking non-stuff. It is the intelligence at the cellular level, the intelligence geneticists primarily locate inside DNA. Life unfolds as DNA imparts its coded intelligence to RNA (ribonucleic acid), which in turn imparts bits of intelligence to the cells and thousands of enzymes, which then use their specific bit of intelligence to make proteins. At every point in this sequence, energy and information have to be exchanged or there could be no building life from lifeless matter. In this perspective it is the intelligence encoded within each cell that allows creation.

The exception and/or rejection of any of these theories cannot avoid recognizing a common thread, *intelligence* and communication *within* the cell.

While there are shared qualities of all cells there are also discernable differences between the types of cells within the body. The cells may all share the same DNA, yet they seem to place more emphasis on certain properties, while minimize others to perform as a specific type of cell. A cell that makes up the eye is different than one that makes up the heart. And yet if these cells are moved during the first six weeks of human development they can adapt to perform the function required of a cell in that environment. In other words, if a cell is removed from say the kidney, and replaced in the larynx, it becomes a fully functioning, identifiable larynx cell.

As adults, we maintain a relatively stable number of cells that make up our body. In spite of constant attrition, elimination and replacement, the overall number remains fairly constant. We are born with a certain number of cells. As these cells are replaced they may be of stronger, weaker, larger or smaller composition.

Some cells apparently may have a greater capacity for change, modification or alteration than others. One type of cell with this capacity for alteration is commonly referred to as a *fat cell*. There are many functions that can be performed by fat cells. Some include protection for internal organs, storage of fluid or nutrients, or insulation. There is a percentage or proportionate amount of fat that is necessary in the human body for healthy, efficient functioning. Percentage and distribution of these fat cells differs between men and women. Women have higher percentages of body fat. This is particularly in the abdominal area (to protect reproductive organs) and in the breasts, which are approximately 50% fat cells.

During our lifetime we experience changes in our growth patterns. We develop rapidly from an infant to an adolescent. By the time we have reached twenty-two years of age we have generally stopped growing in height. It is a commonly held belief that based upon our genetic background, diet and activity levels we will develop a particular body type (size, shape and proportion). These traits will typically resemble other members of our birth family. If being human were simply a mechanical process, then surely this would be the end of the equation.

One has only to visit or observe any public gathering to notice exceptions to this simple formula. The exception is your thoughts. But do your thoughts originate in your brain or in your mind? Many individuals believe that your thoughts originate in your brain. In Western medicine we have and are studying the brain extensively. It is generally agreed upon that the brain is made up of two hemispheres; the right and the left.

The right hemisphere is believed to possess the more creative aspects of a person. Art, music, emotion and spatial perception. The left hemisphere is believed to be more orderly, controlling language, reason and morality.

The right hemisphere of the brain is believed to control the left side of the body, and the left hemisphere is believed to control the right side of the body. At least these are the beliefs held about individuals who are *normally organized*. Perhaps 20% or more individuals are believed to be *reverse organized*. Reverse organized meaning that the qualities believed to be attributed to the right and left hemispheres of the brain are reversed. Perhaps the most important word in any of these previous statements is *believed*.

Psychological Framework

We would like to now introduce you to the concept of mind. A non-physical, yet powerful determinant as to what you will see, what you will feel and what you will do. While the brain is physical, the mind is not.

Let us first make the distinction between the different aspects of the mind. The mind as we define it consists of three separate aspects: *Conscious* mind; *Unconscious* (subconscious) mind; *Collective* (group, higher-self) mind. For the purpose of this writing we shall address only the conscious and unconscious mind.

We begin with the conscious mind. This is the *parental* aspect of your mind. It is a type of *gatekeeper*. It can chose to allow information in, or to deny access. The things that you do are decided by your conscious mind. Or so it may appear. The conscious mind accepts or rejects information based upon whether or not it deems the information valuable or correct. If you are wearing an article of clothing that you believe you look particularly attractive in and receive a compliment on it, you tend to accept the compliment. If on the other hand you are wearing something that you don't particularly like or care for and receive a compliment, you are likely to dismiss it. You may even go a step further and dismiss the credibility of the person offering the compliment all together, including future comments. This is an important principle in the creation of self-concept. We will discuss this further in chapter two.

In either of these cases the conscious mind will pass the information along to the unconscious mind for storage. This is but one of the many important and unique functions of the unconscious mind. In addition to storing and organizing information and memories, the unconscious mind performs a wide variety of tasks. Some of the aspects of the unconscious mind that we utilize in *The Body Contouring Programme*™ include; preservation of the body, and the willingness to follow orders. Dr. Tad James has created a list of twenty tasks or charges of the unconscious mind. You will find this list on page nine of this chapter.

As we begin to understand and accept these premises of the unconscious mind we become able to more effectively and efficiently assist an individual in realizing their desired changes. We can then assist them in releasing and / or modifying outdated beliefs. We can also guide them in constructing and implementing new useful ones. All beliefs that an individual holds are of benefit to them. As a therapist it is your responsibility to allow your client to view these beliefs in a non-judgmental way. As beliefs are uncovered the client then has the opportunity to eliminate, modify or reinforce them. This in turn is when change can begin to take place. Remember, beneath your conscious level of awareness you have all the resources necessary to change yourself. How you perceive yourself is either

Properties of the Unconscious Mind

1. Store memories

2. Domain of emotions

3. Organize all memories

4. Repress memories with unresolved negative emotion

5. Present memories for "rationalization"

6. Keep emotions repressed for protection

7. Run the body

8. Preserve the body

9. To be a highly moral being

10. To be a servant, to follow orders

11. Control and maintain all perceptions

12. Generate, store, distribute and transmit "energy"

13. Respond with instinct and habit

14. Needs repetition for long term projects

15. Programmed to continually seek more and more

16. Does not need parts to function

17. Symbolic

18. Takes everything personally

19. Works on the principle of least effort

20. Does not process negatives

maintaining or creating changes in your body right now. By simply changing your perceptions - how you perceive yourself - you can change your body and your life.

By now you have probably asked yourself either"Yeah, so tell me something I don't already know.", (we hope this is the case) or "Where do you come up with this stuff?". Whether you fall into either category we feel that it is important to reinforce these theories. You can gain greater understanding of both the physiological and psychological aspect by exploring further many of the books listed in the reference section at the end of this text. In spite of the still often controversial concepts addressed here there is an increasing body of research material being presented to offer explanation and support for these theories.

Bodymind

From the formerly held belief of separateness, we will now continue on to discuss the interconnectedness of the mind and body. *Bodymind* is a term that Dr. Candace Pert, director of the brain biochemistry division at the National Institute of Mental Health, has chosen to use to describe the interconnectedness of the mind and body. Dr. Pert writes that as a result of her research DNA appears to be almost as much sheer knowledge as it is matter. This once again offers further support of the presence of intelligence inherent in the cells. With this intelligence the cells communicate with one another. This was at one time thought to be electrical in nature. The more accepted theory now holds the opinion that a simultaneous chemical reaction takes place. However the emerging concept of an immeasurable presence, perhaps best defined as knowledge or intelligence simply occurs, allowing cells to communicate.

If you remember having had a dream or perhaps even a nightmare from which you awoke in a cold sweat, heart pounding, experiencing all of the physical symptoms of fear... as if running or hiding from someone or something frightening. Obviously, you were only dreaming. However, did your body respond to your experience of the dream any differently than it would have responded to your experience of a similar waking event? Your mind's ability to respond to the stimulus presented is phenomenal and nondiscriminatory.

Your unconscious mind is incapable of distinguishing any difference between a very complete accurate visualization and an *actual* event. In other words, the neurology of your body actually experiences -- has the same feeling, fires the same brain synapses -- during a visualization process that it would if experiencing a physical event.

Another example of this is in a study that was undertaken in which three groups of young men played basketball. One of these groups played basketball three hours a day, the second did absolutely nothing to do with basketball and the third group visualized shooting baskets and playing basketball quite intensely. At the end of a number of weeks, they brought the groups back together and found that, in deed, the ones that had been practicing everyday excelled beyond the others. The group who had not played during the test period found their skills lacked considerably compared to either of the other two groups. However, the group who thought about playing basketball and visualized doing it, did virtually as well as those who had been practicing right along. This was not a random group of young men, these were men who had been playing basketball regularly and were athletes in that field.

Energy follows thought and thought follows energy. In our existence as human beings, we are much more than physical bodies and mental processes. Mind and body are inseparable. A basic emotion can be described as a feeling or as a molecule of a hormone.

"Without feeling the feeling there is no hormone; without the hormone there is no feeling. ...There is no pain without nerve signals that transmit pain; there is no relief from pain without endorphins that fit into the pain receptors to block those signals. Wherever thought goes, a chemical goes with it."

- *Ageless Body, Timeless Mind* Deepak Chopra, M.D. (1993) -

According to this model of quantum physics, the world in which we live is being constantly created and renewed through a flow of energy and information. The flow of energy and information is a "two-way street". The form that is manifest through the observation of energy and information is creative reality. *Reality* is what you perceive.

In *Ageless Body, Timeless Mind* Dr. Deepak Chopra points out that man is the only animal that has a concept of aging. Because we are aware of this aging taking place we tend to age more rapidly. As we are aware of our mortality we tend to expedite it. We are generally born with a body capable of exceeding 200 years of age! Indeed, people in Akasia currently live to be up to 165 years of age! This is in part due to their belief in longevity. Their society places a greater value on a long life. In contrast we in the West typically have a life expectancy of somewhere in our 70's. In either case people have a self-fulfilling prophecy. They live roughly as long as they believe is possible.

By the same token, we recover from any experience based upon the beliefs we hold about it. For example: how many times have you cut yourself and had it heal without a scar? Why is it then that some cuts or injuries result in scars? It is because of the belief held about the trauma resulting in scaring. If cells are being replaced in an on-going basis, how do they know to become "scar cells". Some people refer to this as a *cellular memory*. This theory presents the opinion that long after the injured cells have been replaced the memory of the injury continues to exist. It is due to the memory or belief held about the injury that continues to direct the new cells to continue to form in a confused or *out of balance* way resulting from the injury. When we use a technique such as Time Line Therapy™ to reevaluate and modify the beliefs held about an experience we often find that he physical component clears up as well.

Further research has shown that somewhere in our late twenties to early thirties we in the West start preparing to die. The pituitary gland, in response to these beliefs held, begins to limit or eliminate the production of certain hormones. Hormones that when present actually maintain an individual at a much younger *biological age*. The reduction of hormone production can be the start of a very long process, the process of aging, and ultimately, death.

There appears to be an ever-increasing body of knowledge, including this book, which supports the successful reversing of the aging process. People who take an active part in pursuing and valuing their quality of life are often observed to possess a younger biological age and appearance. A wonderful aspect of these findings are that apparently an individual can adopt these techniques and beliefs at anytime in their life and begin to experience an apparent *youthing* process at any point in their life! There seems to be a positive correlation between the practice of these beliefs and technologies and appearance, health and chronological life extension. All of these reports and observations seem to support the existence of Bodymind.

There have been several books written on health, healing and recovery from illness by utilizing mental and physical interactions. There are a seemingly infinite number of self-help and psychology books. Nutrition, diet and exercise books are equally abundant. In the creation of *The Body Contouring Programme*™ we offering the first *pro-active* approach to assisting an individual in accessing and utilizing their individual power in creating significant lasting positive physiological as well as psychological changes.

After reviewing this brief explanation of our view and implementation of the mind-body connection, or Bodymind, let us assure you, the *reality* of the physical changes desired by our clients is readily observably by all.

Chapter Two

Creation, Maintenance and Importance
of Self-Concept/Self-Esteem

One of the most basic needs that an individual has is the desire to feel good about, or at least comfortable with, him or herself. There are several ways in which individuals do this. It may be as simple as looking at their reflection in a mirror. It might be by asking for someone's opinion about something.

Even though we consider ourselves individuals, we tend to accept or value other's opinions as much or more than our own. Indeed our own opinions are the eclectic result of exposure to the opinions or values of others. Our lives are full of constant daily checks and reminders of who we believe we are.

These daily checks are composed of bits of information that we evaluate and scrutinize on either a conscious or unconscious level. We then accept or reject the information based upon our own internal filter system. Two of the major components of this internal system are our self-concept and self-esteem.

Many people use the terms self-concept and self-esteem interchangeably. For the purposes of this program we view the terms as being distinct from one another and define them separately. Also, because such a plethora of information on the subjects are available, we'll keep it brief.

Self-Concept

Self-concept is the **image** you have of yourself. Each of us carries about with us a personal mental blueprint or picture of ourselves. On a conscious level, it may be vague or ill-defined. In fact, it may not be consciously recognizable at all. But it is there, complete. This self-image is your conception of the who/what/why/how you are. It is based upon a relatively stable set of perceptions you hold about yourself. Perceptions that include physical features, emotional states, talents, likes, dislikes, values, roles, philosophical, religious and political beliefs and so on. These perceptions change over time and the different aspects of one person's self-concept may be quite different from that of the aspects of another person's self-concept. Whereas, a significant part of one person's self-concept might consist of social roles, for someone else, it may be physical appearance, friendships, health, accomplishments or skills. It has been created from your own beliefs about yourself... about who you are. Most of these beliefs have unconsciously been formed from past experiences, successes and failures, humiliations, triumphs and the feedback you've received from others, especially in early childhood. From your interpretation of these experiences, you mentally construct a "self" (or a picture of a self). Once an idea or belief goes into this picture it becomes "true", as far as you are concerned. Without questioning its validity, you proceed to act upon it just as if it were true, and in your experience, it is true. The only reality is yours and everything that exists is inside your subjectivity.

While the infant at birth most certainly has a concept of being, it is without a concept of *self* as *human* being. Thus, the infant learns in order to survive in its new world. Just as the puppy learns *dog* being or the bunny learns *rabbit* being.

Shortly after birth, the infant begins to differentiate among the things in its environment, begins to recognize the familiar face, sounds that accompany different things, responses to their own different sounds, each becomes a separate part of the world. Then, at 6 or 7 months of age the child begins to recognize himself as distinct from his surroundings. Rather than staring at a foot or a hand as if they were strange objects, the child seems to suddenly realize, "Hey, this is me." At this very early age, the self-concept is almost exclusively physical. It is, however, social interaction that almost totally creates the self-concept.

As children learn to speak and understand language verbal messages contribute to the developing self-concept. A child has no way of defining self other than through the eyes of surrounding adults so these appraisals have a profound influence on the developing self-concept.

Self-concept is shaped by the minor events in one's life, as well as giant events.

Later in life, the influence of reflective appraisal is less powerful. The evaluations of others still influence beliefs about the self in some areas, such as physical attractiveness and popularity. In other areas the looking glass of the self-concept has become distorted so that it shapes the input of others to conform with our existing beliefs.

For example, if your self-concept includes the element "unattractive" you may respond to a compliment by thinking, "He must need glasses." The case of the child who is labeled "shy" may find him or herself withdrawn or introverted. While in actuality they are experiencing the same feelings and emotions as the average person in any given situation. The only difference is the filter they place upon the emotion or the experience. In this particular situation the behavior is labeled "shy". This label "shyness" is supported by those around him.

To a degree we judge ourselves by the way others see us. We encounter the idea of knowing ourselves through the 'mirrors' of others. You might argue that not every part of your self-concept is shaped by others, but that there are certain objective facts recognizable by self-observation alone. Indeed some features of the self are immediately apparent, but the significance we attach to them depends greatly upon the opinions of others.

We are more than passive recipients of environmental influence. Both consciously and unconsciously we create our environment as well as respond to it. In *The Concept of Self* Kenneth Bergen (1971) describes how social comparison shapes our self-concept. Bergen explains that people have a continuing need to establish the correctness of their beliefs, something that is often difficult because exact standards may be hard to identify. Therefore, people often look at others as a way of judging themselves. They compare their beliefs, attitudes, behaviors and **appearance** with those around them in order to establish the validity of their own perceptions.

We pay a lot of attention to our physical appearances these days. Furthermore, the interpretation of characteristics such as weight or our physical appearance depends on the way people important to us regard it.

Our culture in the United States generally sees fat as undesirable. This is because others tell us so. In a society where obesity is ideal, a person regarded as extremely heavy would be admired. In the country of Brazil, for example, it is generally held that the ideal female figure is pear-shaped. In the same way the significance of being single or married, solitary or sociable, aggressive or passive depends upon the interpretation society attaches to such traits. Thus the importance of a given characteristic in your self-concept reflects the significance we see others attach to it.

In today's society, self-image is greatly influenced by mass media. Periodicals, newspapers and best-selling books offer the latest diet and fitness trends. Television commercials are filled with scenes of slender, happy people. Consequently, we find people berating themselves that they need to lose weight or to begin or intensify a fitness program. More and more people appear to be modeling the so-called beautiful people. In some instances the program utilized in acquiring that perfectly beautiful body becomes at the least excessive, and sometimes borders abusive. In her book *Self*-Esteem, Gloria Steinem (1993) makes the observation that "society's standards for physical perfection seem to be immutable and right, while our bodies are variable and wrong."

Is it any wonder we are sometimes confused about how or why we feel the ways we do about ourselves?

In all the moments, days, months, years of your lifetime there have been other moments resembling this, but none exactly like this one - this one is unique - this one is now. Like each of us, we may search for, cultivate and find similarities with others, but there is only one me and only one you. As communication educator Virginia Satir stated, "There is not another duplicate of yourself in the world, nor has there been in the 74 billion people before you, or the 5 billion that are here now. You are unique... you couldn't possibly compare yourself to anyone else..."

Self-Esteem

Self-esteem is the product of how you <u>feel</u> about yourself; the internal barometer of contentment with the concept you have of yourself.

Self-esteem can be seen as a product of the messages you've received throughout your lifetime. Family is the first place you receive such messages. Family provides us with our first feelings of adequacy and inadequacy, acceptance and rejection. Even before children can speak, people are making evaluations of them.

The earliest months of life are full of messages that shape the self-concept and, ultimately, self-esteem. The amount of time parents allow their children to cry before attending to their needs communicates nonverbally to the children over a period of time just how important they are to the parents.

The parental method of handling infants speaks loudly. Do they affectionately play with the child? Do the parents hold the child close, or treat them like so much baggage? Do they change diapers or carrying out feeding and bathing in a brusque, businesslike manner? Does the tone of voice with which they speak to the child show love and enjoyment or disappointment and irritation?

Most of these messages are not intentional ones. However, nonverbal statements play a big role in shaping children's feelings about being okay or not okay.

You can probably recall someone you once knew who helped enhance your self-esteem by acting in a way which encouraged you to feel special, accepted or worthwhile, appreciated or loved. Now recall someone who acted in either a big or small way to diminish your self-esteem. In either situation, you chose to feel a particular way about that interaction based on your learned perceptions.

To the extent that you have received supportive messages, you have learned to appreciate and value yourself. To the degree that you have received critical messages, you are likely to feel less valuable, loveable and capable.

As you go through life you accept or reject comments and criticism based upon how credible the source of the criticism is, how important the person giving the criticism is to you, and how well the criticism fits into your model of yourself and the world.

How many times have you been told something you felt was inconsistent with your own beliefs, and therefore dismissed it? How many times have you been told something you mightily rejected on an adult, reasoning level, but felt on some internal 'gut' level the comment held true? How many times have you been told something with which you absolutely agreed? In one manner or another, this happens to everyone.

We are what we think we are. We are exactly what we imagine ourselves to be. Extensive research by Prescott Lecky, an educator and one of the pioneers in self-image psychology, sheds enormous light on how we look at 'poor' students. He concluded that typically, almost without exception, poor grades in school are due in some degree to the student's self-conception or self-definition. These students hold ideas that include, "I am dumb," "I am a naturally poor speller," "I am weak in math," "I do not have a mechanical mind," "I am ugly," etc. With such self definitions, the student has to do poorly in order to be true to himself. He literally creates experiences that confirm his beliefs.

Consider, in the case of a young girl who considers herself "ugly", "a little on the heavy side", "clumsy", "flat chested" or even "a poor dancer". The picture she has created as her mental blueprint is fulfilled perfectly as she grows to adulthood. She compliments her own belief by creating more and more experiences that confirm or solidify her "picture" or conception of herself.

Now consider the possibility of changing that blueprint to include all the lithesomeness, agility, sensuousness and beauty she desires. Her very willing and able unconscious mind will create perfectly the physical reality from the plans provided it, just as it has always done.

You now have a pretty good grasp on how it is you've developed your own self-esteem. When you review the "how" of it, keep in mind that no matter what experiences have lead you to feel the way you do about yourself now, you've chosen your feelings. Feelings based upon your learned responses to how others have acted toward you and upon the events in your life -- and that's great! If could choose once, you know you can choose again.

In the words of Leo Buscaglia, "The human mind can imagine both how to break self-esteem and how to nurture it - and imagining anything is the first step toward creating it." We are what we believe we are. In this sense, we and those around us constantly create our self-concepts and ourselves.

Chapter Three

Causes of Limiting Decisions and Beliefs

The beliefs we hold about ourselves are responsible for acceptance or rejection of comments made by others. Some of these beliefs are what are generally considered to be 'positive' beliefs. These beliefs support us in a happy and fulfilling existence. Some beliefs are 'limiting'. They limit us in developing our full potentials. All of our beliefs are of value. They have accompanied us to this point in time where we are ready to consider possibilities.

By identifying and modifying limiting beliefs, we can begin to create and experience an entirely new self-concept. This can often lead to both the setting and attainment of new goals, not the least of which can result in physical changes.

Take for example the woman who was always told that her sister was the pretty one. Or the woman who was constantly told that she would never develop a figure. This can often result in a woman being unable to accept a compliment. This may be due to the woman having created a self-concept that she is undesirable. She becomes unable to accept a compliment which is inconsistent with the beliefs that she holds about herself. This is but one of the possible limiting beliefs addressed in the *Body Contouring Programme*^{TM}.

Individuals hold beliefs that regulate how they view themselves in comparison to others around them. Rita Freedman, Professor of Psychology and Women's Studies, in her book, *Body Love,* reports that in recent studies, the majority of 10 year old girls rated themselves **least** attractive in their school class; teenage girls said they frequently felt ugly; fewer than 50% of college women felt good about their appearance; a majority of adult women considered themselves heavier than they really were as well as heavier than the ideal **they thought** men preferred; and that women considered "pretty" by others considered themselves "plain". The evidence of distorted self-image is other than gender specific. Susan Harter, Ph.D., Professor of Psychology, University of Denver, in another recent study, reports that when considering the average of men, 70% to 90% would want to change something about their appearance; 1/3 would consider cosmetic surgery; more than 1/2 don't like how they look naked.

"I wish I had her figure" is something women have said time after time after time. But why don't you have her figure? There are many reasons behind that statement. In the following pages we will identify some of the reasons for the beliefs we've accepted, either consciously or unconsciously, that have contributed, at least in part, to the shaping of our self-concepts. Most of the reasons cited here can be traced to early childhood development and are presented in that light.

Fear

Fear of causing more attention to be drawn to oneself as they begin to mature and develop physically. Perhaps an uncomfortableness with receiving attention can quite often be an underlying motivation in maintaining a belief that is limiting in nature. It may be a fear of the unknown. It may be fear of change.

In *The Course In Miracles* the opinion is shared that there are only two basic emotions, *Love* and *Fear*. Everything else is a division of these two. And in actuality, fear is the absence of love. There does not need to be a rational basis for this. Indeed, just like in the case of a phobia, the existence of an strongly held irrational belief will create a very strong reaction. In this particular instance, the suppression of physical development.

Here is an example from one of my early clients. In some cultures, societies or families, interaction between younger males and females is very much frowned upon. The idea of having a boy walk their daughter home from school or call them on the telephone in the evening has been something that causes anxiety or tension within the family. As a result of this a young woman may have unconsciously chosen to suppress her physical appearance or development as much as possible in order to deter attention from boys, fearing a negative reaction from her family.

In this case the woman confided that she had always wanted to be beautiful and curvaceous. She was also extremely afraid of how her family would react. She was not allowed to have male friends. This was very hard for her, as she attended a public school with both men and women in attendance.

Eventually her family arranged an engagement for her. She ultimately married, which ended in divorce. Afterwards she sought therapy to achieve freedom from the great guilt and responsibility that she felt for her failed marriage. As she became aware of *her* desires, and recognized the decisions that she had made based upon fear of her families reaction, she was able to modify them. Within a few minutes she had a new attitude towards life. Almost immediately she began to experience physical changes. Over the next few weeks she created the physical body that she had always desired. Last we heard she was happily involved in a relationship, and all was well with her family.

Uncertainty

There is a period of time growing up through adolescence and early teens when people are uncertain of how to act or how to behave. This may be the result of hormonal changes and a rapidly growing and changing body. It may lead to confusion as to how to deal with feelings of awkwardness accompanying such change.

Some individuals exhibit a greater amount of uncertainty or almost preoccupation and concern involved with these feelings. There have been some women appear to have made an unconscious decision along the way to outwardly appear less feminine in order to receive less attention, usually from men and boys, as they were growing up.

Many of these people did originally feel more comfortable with themselves and more comfortable with their interactions with others. However, socially they became able to more comfortably disappear into the wallpaper as it were. From this point they could safely observe rather than outwardly participate in many functions. It could even have to do with a feeling that they weren't as popular as other people or friends. In the case of women, they may have unconsciously suppressed their outward growth and appearance because of this. They began to act out in a socially accepted role as a supporting character, rather than a star.

The confusion as to whether to develop further physically and enter into the limelight, or center of attention became more threatening than the comfort of supporting others. This level of comfort was then related to interaction between the same sex or opposite sex, ending up with the uncertainty as whether to develop further physically. This in turn resulted in stagnating in any further physical development, or even excessive, socially undesirable gain in proportion.

Confusion

A young woman may have had an opinion or belief that "it was in her genes" to become what others might describe as a vivacious or sexy woman. When she did not begin to develop as soon or rapidly as she expected she would, it caused confusion. Since it had not occurred within her perceived appropriate time frame, then perhaps it would not at all. Based upon this confusion she changed her mind and focused on a new outcome. Perhaps she adopted the desire to fit into a more slender mold or athletic build.

Confusion at an early age can often take place with involvement in sports. The girl enjoys sports, yet notices that as other girls begin to develop shapely figures that they are treated differently, or are identified as having different traits, strengths or qualities no longer associated with sports. This could have a lasting effect on maintaining 'athletic' features which might include smaller breasts or a slight, masculine figure.

There could certainly be a combination of more than one issue. However, often this does create a confusion as to whether or not there emerges as what is termed as a more feminine or more athletic build.

Protection / Trauma

Protection from sexual abuse or any type of attention which may have been interpreted as abuse. Choosing not to appear any more developed or any more feminine than possible so as to discourage such treatment. This can often result in excessive weight gain as well. This can be for protection or to help hide the individual within the physical body. Perhaps it's something which has been a long-term problem or on-going pain.

The possibility may exist that there was an early misunderstanding of a behavior. What may have been a harmless, non-threatening behavior may have been misinterpreted, resulting in an undesirable physical development. Even though this behavior may have long since stopped it has left a memory. Based upon that memory a limiting decision or belief has been made. By uncovering this memory and clearly identifying it as a cause, we can modify the behavior stemming from the acceptance of it. This behavior can certainly include physical manifestations.

Unworthiness

A feeling of unworthiness could be the result of a woman at a very young age feeling that she was not worthy or as valuable as others or she was as not deserving of things as other people. This may have been the result of feedback from parents, relatives, siblings. Often times it can be the results of chiding from other people in the family.

Perhaps it was meant to be harmless teasing but outwardly manifested itself in a repression of outward physical manifestation in the woman's body.

It could also be the results of feeling that she could not live up to the expectations placed upon her of constantly trying to obtain something but again feels that she is just not worthy or all the rewards or benefits of being a physically attractive woman. When we uncover these types of beliefs, and eliminate them, the client often begins to experience a whole new life. All of a sudden the things that she was not worthy of become easily attainable. Almost common place eventually. The person feels an increased value of what they are contributing. They in turn begin to contribute more, more in every aspect of their life and those around them.

Reflected Appraisal

Reflected appraisal is the case in which often an individual has created a limiting decision, belief or belief structure installed by the feedback received from people significant in his or her life. Respected others, family members, peers, or perhaps an early boyfriend who may have made comment or reference to the size of a woman's breast or shape or an opinion of what was ideal. Such statements may have been instrumental in creating the woman's self-concept as to what is now her definition of feminine or desirable.

As the woman continues to receive feedback from those around her she identifies with it. The unconscious mind does its part by creating the physical body to respond with the perceptions held. These perceptions may remain at an unconscious level even though the woman's conscious opinion may have changed as to what is acceptable or desirable. The unconscious mind will maintain the earlier decision to keep the body in a certain shape until specific directions to alter this plan is given. This belief may be very strongly held on to, and therefore very resistant to change.

Competition

Competition between family members, sisters and girlfriends. Social competition to see who could appear the most mature or most developed. Who could appear the most feminine. Who could get the most attraction and be the most popular. The results of these interactions often install beliefs that shape the self-concept.

This is something that quite often has been based upon the shape of a woman's figure or the size of a woman's breasts. It could stem from how much attraction they receive from men at early ages. Actually the competition between themselves and others may seem so extreme that the way they choose to cope with the situation is to back out of the competition and allow other girls to take the lime light.

It is also possible that secondary gain may come into play. A young girl may find she receives more attention, albeit expressed as sympathy, from family members or from other friends for her inability to cope with competition.

Typically, awareness of the decision to suppress her physical development is unavailable on a conscious level.

Resentment

Often resentment may begin at a very early age. A girl may have realized the women around her, involved in her upbringing or disciplining her may have been treating her in a manner which she found unacceptable. Because of this she may have chosen to be different than them.

Many times resentment may result from jealousy towards the mother or female figure. If this female figure was full figured or large breasted the girl may have chosen to repress her own physical changes. At some point she may have made a decision, not necessarily a conscious one, to appear as different as possible from the woman she was modeling, actually choosing not to be like her in any way shape or form.

This, in turn, could and does manifest in a completely different physical shape. Often we see this difference between sisters in the same family. Perhaps there was a great deal of rivalry or anger between two sisters. Later in life this is often expressed in statements such as "one woman got all the looks and the other didn't". "My mother and sisters are well-endowed; I just didn't get any". "They were all used up." or "I was just left out".

Role Model

We all grow up grow up identifying with certain people. We may idolize them or use them as role models. Many times there is such a strong desire to identify with or to be like that person we may actually begin to physically resemble that person. We may begin to take on their traits or qualities. Some modeling is done consciously, perhaps in adopting a certain style of dressing, hairstyle, manner of speaking, walking or carrying oneself.

It is also possible to take on or develop the physical features a role model. As in the instance of a young girl whose role model may be a rather petite or small busted woman, she may in fact find her physical development resembles that of her role model. The concept follows, a young person whose role models exhibit physical traits such as being overweight or underweight, balding, prematurely gray hair, of above or below average height, shapely or with all the curves of a piece of lumber, may also develop those same physical traits.

In some instances a girl's role model might have been a man -- a father, uncle, brother, grandfather or a coach. Early on, she may have presented herself as being a *'tomboy'*. Eventually, others express the opinion it is time for her to grow up and she is asked to stop roughhousing with the boys, to dress and act appropriately. No longer allowed to have as much fun as she used to, she may have chosen to repress her outward physical development. Suppressing what might have eventually been considered a more shapely or curvaceous figure that many people would identify as being feminine.

Conclusion

As you can see, all of these limiting beliefs or decisions were made early on in life. Made, quite typically, at a time and age prior to puberty (often prior o age seven), at an age when the body was just beginning to develop. Ultimately, the limiting belief was created concurrent with the making of a decision as to the self-appropriateness of developing any particular physical trait.

Chapter Four

Emotional and Psychological Considerations

In the first three chapters we covered the bodymind, creation and maintenance of the self-concept and self-esteem and the causes of limiting decisions and beliefs. It was no accident we covered these topics in this order. It is our belief we must first have a thorough understanding of a client's mental and emotional state. We need to understand the presenting reason that motivated the client to see` us now. The changes that may need to take place in order to allow the progress and outcome of the desired result. In Chapter Nine, we will specifically address completing an intake to assure both client and therapist are certain of their intentions and outcomes.

First of all, a person who has a well-balanced self-concept and a positive self-esteem tends to view the world in a positive way. We all have the tendency to think other people think as we do. Therefore the individual who feels down, depressed or has a low opinion of him or herself will believe other people see them the same way. They may believe that is the normal way to be, having nothing else with which to compare. This is characterized by the saying "You don't know, what you don't know."

In contrast, an individual with a positive self-concept and self-esteem will tend to feel other people see them favorably and that people in general feel very positive about themselves.

It is therefore our goal in *The Body Contouring Programme*™ to allow our clients the opportunity to create a more positive self-image, self-concept and self-esteem. By developing a positive self-concept they will tend to view themselves more positively, as well as the world around them. People who view their surroundings and the people around them as supportive, positive and encouraging will excel, in general, in other aspects of their lives and specifically, within *The Body Contouring Programme*™.

Exercise

Think of time in your own life when you felt very positive and very supported by those around you. Perhaps there was a task, a project or an objective which seemed to be a bit overwhelming at the time. However, because of the support of those around you and their encouragement, you somehow found yourself with the ability to stay with the task. Whether it was due to your own proficiency or just the feeling of satisfaction when you finally finished the project, there was also quite possibly a certain sense of enjoyment as accompaniment to the completion of the task.

A person nurtured, having the support of those around them and feeling positive about him or herself tends to have more energy and a greater desire to stick with the program and see the end results in a positive light. They will therefore tend to expend more energy upon it, with a greater amount of enthusiasm and devotion to the project.

You may choose to contrast this experience with another time in your life when you felt you were alone or did not have the support of others. Perhaps a time when you felt that there was something you had to do and therefore you may have tended to procrastinate. This might have led you to be somewhat less than compelled to become involved in the project. Ultimately, this can result in less than proficient job performance.

If you were to look back on either one or both of those times or perhaps something going on in your life currently, you may realize that you searched for feedback on your performance. You may tend to feel that other people either reflect the same level of importance or the same amount of triviality towards your project based on your own presentation of the idea.

In contrast, consider something you are excited about. Something you may view as having a positive outcome. Something you desired to do and found those around you were supportive and encouraged you. You may find you feel all people around you are smiling and seeing you in a better light.

That's all well and good for accomplishing a project or a task. Let's look now at your personal opinion of yourself.

We've all had the experience of waking up in the morning and finding we'd just rather stay in bed than get up and face the world ahead of us. Maybe it's because of something that's happened recently or something we feel is imminently on the horizon. Its on days like these we often tend to take a more negative view of everything. Nothing seems to go right. From the way our hair looks to our choice of clothing and the way it fits. Even our physical appearances seem displeasing. This negative appraisal of ourselves may lead to the certainty that other people perceive us the same way.

There are also those mornings we awake excited about something, perhaps something about to happen or something that has just happened. The experience or anticipation has allowed us to feel rather elated. We notice that the people around us respond to us more positively, more encouragingly. Perhaps we see more smiles, more nods, more acknowledgment and acceptance of others. These are days we seem to have more energy or find it easier to accomplish more, accompanied with an overall positive feeling.

Often times we try to duplicate these experiences. Sometimes it is a matter of returning to the same place where we met someone or saying the same things or discussing the same topics. Perhaps trying to recall how we smiled or how we carried ourselves that day, perhaps even going to the extreme of wearing the same clothes we wore on that positive occasion, hoping to repeat it... searching for the one thing we did differently that day. Why was it we felt so positive? Why was it everything fell into place for us? Why was it that no matter what we did everything turned out just right? However, communication is unrepeatable. Whatever has been done, is done; whatever has happened, has happened. Try as we might to duplicate a previous experience, as much and as closely as possible, we'll never do it exactly the same again.

When we hold a positive attitude, others see us more positively. We tend to feel more positive. Some people explain that as dressing for success or dressing good to feel good. Dress the way you'd like to feel. Have the attitude, express the attitude you would like to have. Others may express an opinion that you are just playing or acting.

However, you will find that if you put on clothes you enjoy wearing, put a smile on your face, exhibit a look of confidence while carrying yourself in a confident manner, others will see you as confident. As others perceive you that way and respond to you that way, you will tend to assume those tendencies even more rapidly. And perhaps before you know it, before you even realize it, you have been very confident all day, affecting others in an interactive and a very positive manner. This may sound oversimplified and too easy to believe and yet research shows that, in fact, people who perceive other people as competent are more attractive, more approachable, and more likeable.

Most people also tend to be more attracted to people they perceive as being to some extent like themselves. Think about the people with whom you associate. Stop a moment and think, "Do my friends and associates fully support me in my endeavors?" "Do they have positive outlooks on life?" "Are they enthusiastic and supportive?" Or, are the people you associate with on a daily basis more negative? Do they tend to give more criticism than praise? And, if so, do you find yourself following suit and behaving in much the same manner?

Research shows that a minimum of three positive pieces of feedback or information for each piece of constructive criticism, followed once again by positive feedback and reinforcement produces a fertile environment for change. This is known in certain fields of study as 'sandwiching' feedback. Sandwiching a criticism or an area of improvement between the positive things allows the criticism to be more easily accepted and a suggestion for improvement more easily followed. This technique is also a very productive way to provide feedback for another person in a way in which they know they are doing well.

Contrast this concept to the way many of us were brought up: simply being told we'd done something wrong and being reminded, often repeatedly, that we had done something wrong. Sadly, even our educational system promotes this attitude. We are told how many things we've missed rather than how many things have been done right. Perhaps, if we received a 78% on a test it amplifies the fact that we missed 22, rather than that we were correct on 78.

Western society is largely dependent upon finding fault or fixing blame. Putting others down to make ourselves feel better. You have probably experienced this yourself at some time in your life. Someone tells you how poorly you've done or how that was "bad" or how you "should" have done something else. Consider how very different that is from giving praise on the occasion you did something extraordinarily well, or, even giving you praise and positive feedback for things simply done proficiently and competently, even things that might have been expected of you.

Positive feedback is often reciprocal. Thank someone for opening a door or for pouring a cup of coffee. You'll quite often get a little smile or a twinkle in the eye; an acceptance; a positive feeling.

We've probably all come in contact with people who, whenever we see them, have a smile on their face and something positive to say. We enjoy being around those people. These are the people that support us. These are the people we often seek out when we're feeling down. These are the people that offer inspiration to us.

We are also quite aware of those persons who consistently give us negative feedback and criticism. In spite of our best efforts we realize that all we're going to get from them is negative response. There are even some people who, even were we acknowledged as having created world peace, put an end to world hunger or created a new vaccine that would immunize against any type of illness, that in spite of all those great accomplishments, that person would still say to us, "Well, why did you go about doing it THAT way?"

What we are emphasizing here is choices. The advantage of choosing to have a positive outlook. We all have choices every day. We choose moment to moment. We choose to be at cause in our lives, or conversely, effected by the people and situations presented in our lives. Many people go through their entire lifetimes being 'at effect'. They always have a reason why they couldn't do something. They were unable to do this or unable to do that because, because, because..... If only I had.... Such and such made me.... I couldn't do that because....

If we turn that around and go from the effect to the cause side of the equation and find that quite possibly we allowed someone to stifle us; or that we allowed ourselves to be sidetracked;... we may find we gave away the gift of being responsible for our own lives.

So where does this all lead us? In reviewing the basic model of cause and effect, consider that when we find ourselves at cause in our lives, we find that we are in complete control and that we are, in fact, responsible... and what does responsible mean? It means we are capable of making a response and that, as human beings, we choose our responses. That simple.

Some people will go so far as to accept responsibility for everything, including the rush hour traffic on the freeway. That may seem a little farfetched. However, those people truly feel they are at cause and responsible for their lives. When you meet such a person you may find they are very positive, very motivational. You may not realize right off what it is about them, but there is something you like. Perhaps its just a sense that they really like themselves... and they're responsible for that, too!

In our society it has also become acceptable for us to put ourselves down. To get down on what we've done or how poorly we've done, how we've failed to accomplish something. Whether it was to get that promotion, or that new car or the grades in the class. It is quite acceptable for us all to put ourselves down. In some respects and in some instances, its almost expected.

However, turn that around for a moment. Think of how acceptable it is for you and when the last time it was that you really felt good about something you had done. Something you had accomplished. Rather than expressing how pleased you were with yourself and how proficient you were and what a good job you had done, did you downplay your accomplishment or make some sort of excuse for your proficiency?

Personal put-downs such as "Well, it was because of the other people involved with the project that it turned out so well." "Anybody could have done that." "I just happened to be in the right place at the right time." have become socially acceptable.

If you've ever had the experience to work with professional models or professional athletes, quite often people feel they have a rather cocky, snobbish or "stuck-up" attitude. Often that is because of conversations where someone may say, "You did a wonderful job of that." And they will respond with, "Yes, I know." They are very confident. They accept your praise and they realize that it is true... they accept that as a truth. They see themselves as very competent. They know they are very good at what they do. Unlike many people who may downplay a compliment these people openly grasp these compliments. They accept and own them. You may feel they are rather stuck on themselves because they acknowledge positive things about themselves. And yet, isn't that the way?

Exercise

An exercise in which you might care to participate now or at a later date, or use with future clients is offered here. Ask your clients to make a list, in writing, of ten positive things they like about themselves. Now, it has been our experience that if asked to write down ten things they don't like about themselves, that's often quite an easy task. They may say they could write 20 or 25 just as easily. Next, ask them to write 10 things they actually like about themselves. You may find this is quite often more difficult. Its very easy for other people to see things or to present 10 things they like about someone else, but to actually own that themselves and say, "Yes, I like these things about myself." is a very valuable exercise. You may want to expand on that and go for 20 or 25 things you like about yourself. If that starts to be a bit too difficult you might think about someone you admire or respect or who's company you enjoy and start off by writing 10 things you like about them. And, then look at that list and try that on yourself and find out if you like those same ten things about yourself. Or, are there more things you like about yourself than what's on that list. Or, are there things on that list that do not apply to you.

Once again, we tend to enjoy and like people whom we perceive as being like ourselves, whether its the style of clothing they wear or the way their hair is styled, it could be their choice in music or the type of car they drive or the books they're reading. The person who feels they have very few friends or are rather shy or introverted, may pause for a moment and look for what it is they portray or express nonverbally in their lives. If they find themselves being unapproachable, perhaps they'd care to look at what it is about someone they consider approachable that is different. Does that person exhibit characteristics they'd like to try on? Ask what would happen if they were to do those things themselves.

Exercise

Find someone you admire, someone you have a positive feeling about and make a list of the things you like about them and see how many of those traits you possess and how you would go about possessing the others, should you choose to. You may find that if you begin to wear the style of clothing that you truly would like to wear you may start feeling, acting or responding to yourself in different ways, as well as finding others responding to you in a way that you would like to be responded to. Just a simple change at first perhaps. Remember, confidence and acting... if need be, act the part of the person you'd like to be until you, in fact, become the person you want to be.

We talked about self-esteem in Chapter One. We realize that we are the eclectic result, quite often, of the reflective appraisal of people around us. These basic beliefs and traits were established somewhere between or prior to the age of 4-7. As John Piaget, the child psychologist says, "If you think back to when you were 4-7 years old, were you capable of making the types of decisions you would make today about your life?" Think about that for a moment. Would you or your client like to have a 4-7 year old come in and outline what they expect of you in your life, what they would like for you to do, how you should act or interact with others? Perhaps not. What we would offer to you is that you take the opportunity to really look at who you would like to be now. Make a very conscious decision about that and look at the types of behaviors you've displayed over the years. Ask yourself, "When did I decide to behave this way?" "Am I doing this because someone else felt that was an appropriate way to behave?" Ask yourself what will happen if you change. What would you be giving up? What would you be gaining? Are you willing to do that now? You may find that the more positive self-image you have, even if it at first seems to you a bit unnatural or a bit copied, modeled, stuck-up, that as you get into playing that role, it becomes more comfortable to you. You may, in fact, find that other people respond to you quite differently. Particularly, people who have been putting you down along the way or people who have been stepping on you or people who have been trying to feel better about themselves or their own shortcomings by pointing out yours. You may find you meet a whole new caliber of friends or colleagues. You may even start going places where you would actually like to be rather than places you've been going because other people you associated with go there.

The client that comes to you, or perhaps, you yourself, are studying this type of work because you desire to have a change in your life. You desire to have a better life. Realizing that, as pointed out earlier, if everything was going just perfect in your life, then you would have very little motivation to change.

It is doubtful you'll see a client come in and say to you, "You know, I have the perfect relationship and I'm making the perfect amount of money and I'm getting the right amount of exercise and feedback and esteem from others. I feel absolutely wonderful every place I go and in everything I do." If they do come in like that and are congruent, you might just ask them how exactly they do that. We will discuss NLP later in Chapter Five. You will want to learn their strategy and how to install it in yourself and in others.

Other than that hypothetical individual who may or may not ever come into your office, you want to learn from that and think for a moment what it is that you, or ask your client what it is that they would like to possess; what they really want out of life; what they're willing to give up to have that, if, in deed, anything.

Our behavior may be perceived as positive or negative or perhaps, best of all, simply of value.

Consider that most people feel they can identify two basic categories of experiences within their lives. They either have 'good' experiences or 'bad' experiences. Now, good experiences are things that most people would like to repeat. Such as revisiting a restaurant where they had a good time, or perhaps, having spent pleasurable time with somebody, choosing to spend time with them again. Perhaps they bought a particular make of car, had very good luck with it and would buy that make of car again. Those are all 'good' experiences and may be considered experiences worth repeating.

On the other side of that, perhaps you went to a restaurant at which you had a less than enjoyable time or you went out with someone whose company you did not enjoy or you bought a particular make of car with which you had a great deal of trouble. Many people would view those as 'bad' experiences.

However, I would like to pose this possibility to you... this alternative or option. The 'good' experiences are things you choose to do again and the 'bad' experiences are typically events or a chain of events you've chosen not to repeat. You might actually consider that you've learned from what you've previously called bad experiences. Having learned from them you've chosen not to repeat them. Some people would say you are learning from your mistakes. While this is true, I would ask you to evaluate learning as a good thing or a bad thing. Most people would choose to put learning in a positive category since learning is, in fact, a good thing. So if you're having bad experiences, which are actually learning experiences, you might want to recategorize them as having good experiences and learning experiences. If you find that works for you, as most people do, you may realize that since learning is a good thing, you are actually having good experiences and good experiences. So, what it all boils down to is that you are only having good experiences.

So, how would you choose to respond to your experiences? Positively? We hope so. Because you realize that all of your experiences are good experiences. It would seem rather self-defeating to have experiences other than that. Particularly when they are all positive, good experiences. When you view the world this way and others this way and all of your experiences this way, you will find that you are responding to the world in a positive way. People in turn will respond to you in a positive way. Even your opinions of others will become more positive. Such is the spiral of you thinking positively and seeing people positively and they seeing you positively and allowing changes to take place.

Changing your beliefs or how you view and interpret your experiences might be just as easy as changing your mind. By simply recategorizing an experience or series of experiences, a gestalt of experience, you may find you've had a very wonderful life. As well, you may find that often just presenting this reframe to a client can be very empowering, particularly for people who feel they were constantly having 'bad' experiences. Soon your clients begin to realize they are having nothing but good experiences, are making choices in a positive light and finding it much easier to accept having a wonderful life. The option offered you and your client now is that you can just change your mind.

Those of you who have a background in Neuro Linguistic Programming, interpersonal communication or human communication may be quite familiar with this theory and yet it is a concept that certainly bears repeating since, after all, redundancy does improve accuracy. We'll discuss specific utilization of repetition in *The Body Contouring Programme*™ more fully in Chapter Nine.

Exercise

As you take these steps now to create a more positive self-esteem, you may find it is just as simple as viewing the world from a positive perspective. Take a moment, whenever you have an opinion, an evaluation you might make of someone or something, and pause to determine whether that opinion or evaluation is based on a belief you've chosen to hold. Where did it come from? Whose belief was it before it was yours? Does it serve you? Has it served you well in the past? If so, hold onto it. Should you find, however, you want to alter or change that view or interpretation, you may discover you are now infinitely more capable of making your own decisions about what it is you choose to believe. You may discover you are capable now of basing your beliefs on what is actually happening before you rather than on an experience you had in early childhood or on an opinion expressed by someone else who was, perhaps with good intentions but otherwise misguided.

We often hear people proclaim they are products of their environment or their upbringing. Certainly, to an extent, we agree. We also realize to say that is ALL we are or can ever be relegates us to a position of suspended animation. Today, we have incredible resources at hand to aid us in generating an environment conducive to the emotional and physical well-being of all of us.

There is infinitely more knowledge available now in the fields of self-concept, self-image, psychology and human behavior than was available during most of our parents' time. Even in the bookstore where you may find a copy of this book, you will notice the self-help and psychology, the health and fitness sections are prolific with titles of books written on these subjects. Concepts and attitudes found only among a very small minority 20 or 30 years ago are now available for general consumption.

"We can consider the process of healthy growth to be a never ending series of free choice situations, confronting each individual at every point throughout his life, in which he must choose between the delights of safety and growth, dependence and independence, regression and progression, immaturity and maturity."

-Abraham Maslow-

When considering the possibilities and options offered here, consider, if you will, the following Random House Dictionary (1980) definition: Revision - "re-", a prefix meaning: again or anew; "vision", noun meaning: 1. the act or power of seeing; 4. an imaginative conception or anticipation.

Consider taking another look at the concept you have of yourself. You created it. You can re-vision it.

This book is an effective result of our exposure to many different theories. In sifting through, reviewing, testing and utilizing these varied theories and concepts, we have found that in accepting the basic premises of quantum mechanics; understanding how you have created your self-concept; how your self-esteem, in whatever condition it is in, is the product of your conception of yourself and the beliefs, both supportive and limiting, you hold about yourself and by considering the possibility of revisioning it all, you've taken the first and largest step to change. What we offer you are resources and techniques with which to effect the change you desire. As always, the choice is yours.

It is not a matter of deciding on whether or not to use your imagination. You already do. You see, you do, you are. Constantly and continuously. It is simply a matter of now consciously deciding what it is you choose to imagine and create.

II

Development
of

The
Body
Contouring
Programme™

Chapter Five

Hypnosis, NLP and Time Line Therapy™

Hypnosis, trance, visualization, guided imagery or focused attention, the names may vary based upon the context in which individuals may chose to use them. However, for the purpose of this book, please feel free to use them interchangeably, we do. Remember...meanings are in people, not in words.

Hypnosis

Hypnosis is perhaps one of the most misunderstood terms and techniques in the area of therapy. Hypnosis, by definition is "*A focused state of attention*". In actuality it is a naturally occurring state. We all go in-and-out of trance as a part of our daily lives.

The actual word "hypnosis" is from Latin, *hypnos*, meaning sleep. This was the term that James Braid coined to describe the technique that he used. The only connection that sleep had to do with the process was that the patient had their eyes closed. This was a highly effective, yet unnecessary, technique to allow the patient to focus their attention on the suggestions being given. With their eyes closed the patient was free from visual distractions as well as better able to visualize or imagine the suggestions being offered. People who do not understand the concept of hypnosis have long believed that it is a process that is done to you. Even today many people still hold this belief. Unfortunately some individuals who openly admit to using hypnotic techniques believe that it is something that they do to the client. However, the fact of the matter still is that *all hypnosis is self-hypnosis.*

The world famous Franz Anton Mesmer utilized hypnotic suggestion to assist his patients in recovery. While it is true that Mesmer felt that he was using *Animal Magnetism* to assist in healing people, he was actually using suggestion. Mesmer constructed elaborate devices to pass over individuals. He even created tanks to immerse them in. Ultimately he had refined his devices so well that he was able to "Mesmerize" entire areas. Patient needed only to visit these sites to become miraculously healed.

As Mesmer's reputation spread, so did his success. In fact he was so successful at treating his patients that the other physicians of the day demanded that the French government establish a board of inquiry into his methods. Unfortunately the board's findings were that "They could *see* nothing going on in Dr. Mesmer's treatments". Based upon these findings the popularity of Mesmer diminished. He was labeled a fraud. The people of his day returned to the "modern" medical practices.

What Dr. Mesmer was actually doing was allowing individuals to utilize their own innate healing ability to take place. Unfortunately then, just as today, most people placed the ability to heal themselves in the hands of someone else. Mesmer's reputation as being revolutionary and highly successful had allowed individuals to visit him and become healed (healing themselves) through his processes.

This is still very obvious today. The use of placebo drugs is found to be successful in treatment 40%-60% of the time. This is a definite example of hypnosis. By believing that something will happen and then experiencing it. Focusing attention on the desired outcome, while holding a strong belief in the process necessary for it to occur.

Hypnosis itself is a very scientific process. There are three very basic and necessary components for hypnosis to occur. The individual must be intelligent, imaginative and have desire.

The individual must possess enough intelligence to understand the suggestions of the therapist. They must be able to focus their attention and concentrate on the voice of the therapist. Actually, contrary to popular belief, the more intelligent an individual is, the easier they are to hypnotize. They find it quite easy and relaxing to follow and / or implement suggestions.

In order to be hypnotized an individual must have an imagination. They must be able to create a picture to associate with the suggestions. In fact the word *imagine* means "to make a picture". I would like to point out at this time that this has been a long held and highly accepted belief. However the most current research supports the findings that individuals can experience suggestions in unique ways. This may be an individual creating a feeling or sound in order to interpret a suggestion. In any case the experience is valid for the individual.

There is no right-way or wrong-way to experience or participate in hypnosis. There is only the individual's personal experience of it. We are all individuals, with individual values and experiences. To compare ourselves with others is just that, a comparison. Again, there is no right-way or wrong-way, there is just the experience.

The desire that an individual has may vary. They may desire to work with one therapist, but not another. They may desire to work on one area but not another. In any case an individual **will not** perform any suggestion during or after hypnosis that they are not desirous of. In other words, a person's values do not change during or as a result of hypnosis unless it was their specific desire to do so prior to the hypnosis session.

This is what doctors rely upon when they suggest that you "take these pills and you'll feel better in the morning". As a patient you have a desire to feel better, so you follow the suggestion and typically feel better in the morning. However, often the patient who is not confident in the doctor will take the pills, not believing that the doctor really grasped how the patient was feeling, and will therefore not receive the same benefit from the treatment as the patient who was confident in the doctor.

By the same token a dentist may suggest that "you will feel a *slight* discomfort". This suggestion is used to predispose the patient to experience what the dentist felt was appropriate rather than creating a potentially greater experience of discomfort that the patient may attribute to the experience.

In 1958 the American Medical Association AMA sanctioned the use of hypnosis. This was probably done without their conscious awareness that they have always employed it within their practice of medicine.

On the other side of the coin, there have been a few areas in the world that have enacted laws to determine who may legally practice hypnosis. It is unfortunate that the agencies governing these practices often have little or incorrect knowledge about hypnosis. As a result those areas may suffer due to the limited availability of qualified hypnotherapists.

Neuro Linguistic Programming - NLP

Neuro Linguistic Programming (NLP) has been described as *"A trail of techniques - leading to specific outcomes."* This over simplification leaves out many aspects of NLP, including the importance of language. The combination of both use and interpretation of the language being used is studied and identified. The creation and development of NLP may possibly be one of the greatest tools to be made available to therapists this decade.

The field of NLP was originally developed by Richard Bandler and John Grinder in the early 1970's. Much of their fundamental work was based upon observing some of the greatest therapists of our time. Individuals such as Virginia Satir, Fritz Perls and Dr. Milton Erickson were observed and modeled. Through a compilation of the work of these and other individuals, similarities and differences emerged.

As the techniques used were identified they were cataloged. After cataloging they were taught. After being taught they were observed for effectiveness. Beyond this they were modified for maximum effectiveness.

The NLP term used for this process is modeling. The basic concept of modeling is observing greatness; determining the process used; installing or teaching the process to others.

Modeling is but one small aspect of the overall body of knowledge contained within the field of NLP. It is however an important one that we utilize in *The Body Contouring Programme*™.

Another aspect of NLP is the techniques developed to determine how a person views or relates to the world around them. This includes determining and utilizing a person's lead and primary representational system.

The basic NLP model recognizes individuals as having visual, auditory and kinesthetic traits. There is certainly much more to it than this. However, this is the basic model.

By thoroughly understanding and utilizing these techniques a therapist can rapidly assess a client's model of the world. By understanding and relating to a client's model of the world a therapist can then assist the client in realizing the greatest and fastest change.

Have you ever met someone who you instantly seemed to like. This can often be the result of establishing rapport on an unconscious level. This same level can often be obtained by a therapist effectively utilizing techniques taught in NLP trainings.

Perhaps you can recall a time when you met an individual that you felt less than comfortable with, or seemed less than competent. This could most definitely be described as a lack of rapport.

In either of the preceding examples through proper training a therapist can become aware of the individuals preferences. The awareness of these preferences allows the therapist to rapidly gain rapport with the client. Gaining rapport then allows the therapist to assist the client more rapidly.

One of the most powerful aspects of NLP is the specific understanding and use of language. As you gain mastery of language and language patterns you become able to acknowledge as well as assist clients in manifesting personal change. We could spend chapters and even books on this aspect of NLP alone. This information is available from many other sources.

As we have pointed out the body of knowledge within NLP is quite large. The field is growing constantly. There are probably several hundred books either specifically on or closely related to NLP. I would recommend that you read as many as you can. You might want to strongly consider contacting the American Board of Neuro Linguistic Programming (ABNLP) for a list of trainers in your area. If you are not already a certified NLP practitioner and have plans on working with clients then receiving the training will prove invaluable.

Several well-known individuals and techniques have emerged out of the study of NLP. One of the most powerful that we have been exposed to is Time Line Therapy™.

Time Line Therapy™

Time Line Therapy™ was developed by Dr. Tad James and Dr. Wyatt Woodsmall. In 1988 they published their first book on the subject titled *Time Line Therapy and the Basis of Personality.* The initial work that is introduced and outlined here is unfortunately the only book currently available on the techniques. However, trainings in this technique are becoming available on a regular basis throughout the world.

There have been other individuals who talk about time lines, or walk on time lines. These differ from the quite effective techniques of Time Line Therapy™. A primary distinction between the similarly titled techniques, as expressed by Dr. James, is that in Time Line Therapy™ the therapist works with the client, rather than "doing to" a client.

A basic premise of Time Line Therapy™ is that we all store time and memories in a unique way. In spite of our uniqueness, these memories of particular emotional natures are all connected in a type of *gestalt*. The root of this gestalt is a *Significant Emotional Event (SEE)*. When a client is instructed correctly, they can create a *universal timeline* experience. From this timeline the memories may be stored or experienced in a mental or physical way. These memories may be from this lifetime, a pastlife, or passed down genetically. As the root cause of a feeling is discovered, it can be modified or eliminated very rapidly.

The techniques and processes used in Time Line Therapy™ are by far the most effective that we have seen, heard of or experienced. The techniques are in many cases the only remedies that we are aware of for rapidly removing many limiting decisions or beliefs. It has a unique capacity for *future pacing* an individual, so that a trained therapist can gather immediate feedback on the success and completion of the changes being made.

The field of Time Line Therapy™ is rapidly expanding. In order to fully benefit from the most current technology in the field we would strongly recommend that if you plan on working with clients in order to assist them with change that you become a certified Time Line practitioner.

Conclusion

We started this chapter with hypnosis. This is perhaps the oldest form of therapy. We then progressed to NLP, which quite possibly contains the most technical and widely useable techniques. This was followed by Time Line Therapy™, which addresses more specific approaches to change. All of these techniques contain aspects of one another. They are all highly effective and are capable of producing reliable results. It is the mastery and utilization of these techniques that has afforded us virtually 100% success with our clients.

If you plan on using the techniques contained within this book to work on clients, please strongly consider attaining a level of mastery before doing so. We regret not being able to present more detail on these techniques. However, it would be impossible to cover all of the material adequately without writing several volumes. Fortunately there are numerous books written on Hypnosis and NLP. Many are listed in the reference section of this text.

When we began our work in hypnotherapy back in 1974 there were very few schools available to teach even basic hypnosis. As greater acceptance of the field grows so do the number of institutes that offer programs and specialized fields of study. *The Body Contouring Programme*™ has emerged as one of these specialized fields of study.

If you intend to seek a therapist to work with you on your personal changes check for their credentials. If at all possible seek out a *Body Contouring Programme*™ practitioner. Should you as an individual or therapist wish to pursue certification as a *Body Contouring Programme*™ practitioner you would be required to fulfill the following certifications: 1 - certified hypnotherapist and current member of a widely recognized hypnotherapy organization; 2 - certified practitioner of NLP and member of widely recognized organization; 3 - certified Time Line Therapy™ practitioner and current member of the Time Line Therapy™ Association, 4 - certificate of completion from *The Body Contouring Programme*™ seminar, 5 - submittal of 10 successful case histories.

We hope that those of you who are interested in assisting clients will pursue these courses of study. If you have already done so, congratulations! If not, you will find that mastery of these techniques will provide for the greatest change for your client and the most efficient use of both of your time.

Chapter Six

Theory

Typically, individuals considering cosmetic surgery are dissatisfied with one or more aspect of their lives. They are seeking a positive change in the quality of their life. In the case of physical change it will often include grooming habits, components of their diet, types and quantity of exercise and at an ever-increasing rate, elective cosmetic surgery. Some of the procedures regularly performed include: face-lifts; nose restructuring; liposuction and silicone, saline or collagen implants.

Altering the shape, contours or changing the physical appearance of an individual is something that plastic surgeons have been doing quite effectively and successfully for many years. As recently as 1990 over 90,000 women in Southern California alone had silicon breast implants. Recently the opinion has been given, and more widely accepted, that silicone implants are definitely not the alternative to be utilized in attempts to alter the existing physical appearance. This was one of the reasons that our program has been developed and widely accepted. This avoidance of the traditional method of breast enlargement has added to the search for more acceptable and safer, alternatives to breast enlargement.

Unfortunately the majority, if not all, of these surgical practices and procedures have their drawbacks. Even more disappointing is the existence of large volumes of research in existence that presents the findings that the typical client who has had cosmetic surgery will eventually have additional surgeries. This is clear indication the person's needs are unfulfilled.

Individuals utilize these surgeries in an attempt to patch up perceived deficiencies in their lives. These deficiencies may often be the result of low self-concept and/or low self-esteem.

That is not to say the only reason people consider cosmetic surgery is because of poor self-concept or self-esteem. However, there is strong indication that additional review of other aspects of the individual's life could stand to be evaluated in the event that they are seriously considering cosmetic surgery as an option.

The overall motivation that drives the individual to seek cosmetic surgery needs to be soberly addressed. What is the 'presenting' issue that the individual is seeking to fulfill or overcome? How do they perceive their life changing as a result of the surgery? Why is it that they do not experience those things now? Do they currently feel that they are in control of their life, or do they feel that their life is the result of external (including physical) factors?

Does electing to undergo surgery give them a greater feeling of power and/or control over/in their life? The answer to this question is yes. Whether or not the individual is consciously aware of it, the answer is still yes. As a matter of fact control is one of the three major premises that people are motivated to communicate.

Control, affinity, and affection are basic human needs. Control; to have a sense or feeling of personal power or control over issues in their life. Affinity; the desire to be recognized as belonging with an individual or group. Affection; to feel loved, accepted or important by others.

These are three of the most basic needs of a human being. To seek them out is only natural. Attainment of these feelings as virtually an intuitive drive. It is certainly understandably why an individual would seek to take whatever action they deemed necessary to fulfill these basic needs. Elective cosmetic surgery has become a readily available and acceptable avenue for hundreds of thousands of individuals in search of an increased sense of control in their life. A desire for control that they may be consciously or unconsciously aware of.

The choice of undergoing elective cosmetic surgery does allow the individual a measure of control in their life. Unfortunately it also forever relegates them to the underlying reality that they required the assistance of someone else to create and provide them with their desired changes. The reminder of their life they may continue to reflect upon their successes and perceived failures based upon the work of a surgeon.

In contrast, *The Body Contouring Programme*^{TM} has been developed to assist the individual in achieving results comparable or even exceeding the overall physical results of surgery. Through the use of the techniques in *The Body Contouring Programme*^{TM} an individual learns techniques to modify the concepts held in the unconscious mind. Through modifying the previously held limiting decisions or beliefs the individual is empowered to make the changes their self. In the case of physical change it offers a constant daily reminder of the power of the individual.

When individuals become aware of the option to take responsibility and charge of their own lives, and are given techniques, procedures and processes to do so. Their motivation intensifies and they express excitement in implementation of these techniques. By putting the individual in touch with his or her own needs, desires, motivations, feelings of accomplishment, value and worth, the procedures and processes presented here have lead to positive changes in the overall quality of life.

The Body Contouring Programme™ has been designed for the individual who has made a decision to effect some physical change. Physical change that begins with a revisioning of the self-concept and results in enhanced self-esteem.

For many years individuals have utilized hypnosis as a technique for weight reduction. In the late 1960's hypnosis was first studied for breast enlargement. Limited studies have been done infrequently since that period of time. One thing that all the studies had in common is that there was always a high degree of success. However, there was no clear delineation as to how similar the techniques used were.

We often say to a client, weight is only a number. Keeping this in mind we find that when the client responds to wearing a size 11 or a size 9 or a size 3, and if that in fact is their goal, that the issue of whether they weigh 100 pounds, 105 pounds or 155 pounds is no longer an issue. If they feel good and they look good then they have their outcome.

In the mid to late 1980's much work began in the field of liposuction. One of the side affects of liposuction was that many, perhaps as many as 40%, of the individuals receiving liposuction experienced enlargements in their breasts.

In our research we made the intuitive connection that the residual fat cells in the body after liposuction were increasing in size after the procedure had been performed. This is the hypothesis which we developed. We worked under this hypothesis and our results reflect that not only did the breasts respond and increase in size more rapidly, but also more consistently. In addition we have documented significant reduction in the size of the hips, thighs and buttocks when such a change was desired by the client.

In the original body contouring study which is contained in chapter 5 you will note there is less than a 5 pound fluctuation in weight of the body. This was with no specific suggestion given for weight reduction. It has been our experience that the issue of weight is really not the core or prime concern. The prime concern is actually body size, shape and proportion as opposed to weight.

Our experience has been that through a process of creating an ultimate visualization of what the individual would look like is indeed what is in assists them in realizing their outcome. By having the client create a very specific, a very detailed intricate visualization of themselves, a model that depicts every aspect of themselves, from every angle, top, bottom, front, back, side, and then create a technique for having a inward view, such as the metaphysical mirror (this is illustrated later in the scripts), the client creates a very solid connected representation of themselves.

We have found that a state of dissonance is created between the unconscious and conscious mind when the personal image the individual holds differs from his or her actual physical appearance. The unconscious mind then strives and actually has a charge or an obligation to create the physical body to coincide with the image held and the self-concept at that point in time. Therefore it is extremely important to fully associate the client with the image they held of themselves using as many sensory channels as possible, visual, auditory, kinesthetically. To have a solid internal representation system of validation. It is important to incorporate all of the sensory channels of the client for a real, complete and compelling change to occur. The more realistic, compelling and associated visualization you assist your client in creating in their mind the more complete and rapid the change will be.

Hypothesis

We theorized that if we could use hypnosis to reduce the size of the body or weight loss and increase the breast size through mammary augmentation in hypnosis, then perhaps we could make the connection of reducing certain specific parts of the body or enlarging the breasts simultaneously .

Hypnosis and visualization is proven to be quite effective in reducing the size and weight of individuals. Hypnosis and visualization is also effective in increasing breast size. Breasts are approximately 50% fat cells. By altering the size, shape and/or quantity of fat cells, or moving the fat cells, or by replacing the fat cells, and by allowing the individual the opportunity or the option of where to place the amount and/or proportion in size of these fat cells, that the individual should in fact be able to change the contour or shape of their body by relocating the fat cells into or out of the area which their presence would be most desirable.

History

Comparable physical results are achieved through *The Body Contouring Programme™* as opposed to invasive surgeries by utilizing what is possibly the oldest form of healing, through mental processes. *The Body Contouring Programme™ is* the result of combining hypnosis, physiology, self-esteem, communication, Neuro Linguistic Programming and Time Line Therapy™.

We placed our hypothesis into a research project and found that by combining our technique of hypnosis and visualization, using Neuro Linguistic Programming and specific language patterns, our clients did respond faster and with greater results than any previous research that had been conducted in the area of breast enlargement through the use of hypnosis. The results demonstrate virtually 100% success in increasing breast size and shape in clients desirous of such changes.

The results of this research is found later in this text in Chapter Seven on the original research on *Body Contouring™*. The average increase in breast size was approximately 2.25", equivalent to one or more cup sizes. However, participants have experienced and maintained increases in excess of over 4 " in breast size.

The majority of these increases took place within a period of 5 to 10 weeks. It is important to note that this was a process of visualization, there was no specific diet or physical exercise program involved. It has been theorized that if either one or both of these additional regiments were followed along with *The Body Contouring Programme*^{TM} techniques that perhaps even greater or faster results could be obtained.

In response to questions about lasting results, there has been no report of any reversal of any goal which had been obtained. As far as the overall theory goes, that's all well and good, but one of the concerns of *The Body Contouring Programme*^{TM} is the client's self-concept.

Often cosmetic surgery can be quite beneficial. Particularly on a physiological level. However, individuals can often use their own resources, their own power, their own mind to create the same changes, and quite often more, within their own body. Through this process the individual changes not only their physical body, but improves their self-esteem as well.

This also empowers the individual to realize that if they are feeling less of themselves because they do not have the ideal or perfect figure, the one that society is currently dictating, that by changing it, they can change anything. This puts them at being the cause of their changes, rather than being at the effect of an outside source creating the changes. After all, it's their body, and their life.

You can change your body by thinking about it. Putting your thoughts in a more positive direction and feeling more positive about yourself in every aspect of yourself every day will elicit a change. By doing this you empower every aspect of your life. Something that you have created individually. Empowerment that you can carry out into relationships and into the work place. This in turn will effect your social life and has an effect on everyone's life who you ultimately come in contact with.

The Body Contouring Programme™ has been developed to address these areas of self-esteem in conjunction with the elimination of limiting decisions and beliefs, as well as allowing the creation of the more outwardly noticeable physical changes. Thereby addressing the total needs of the individual.

These are the particular reasons that we developed *The Body Contouring Programme*™, to empower the individual. Many people are aware that if you hang out a sign that says "self esteem repaired", quite often you will have very few takers. However, as we look at the statistics on cosmetic surgery you will find that there is a waiting list of people to have this type of work done, and yet they are capable of doing it themselves.

Conclusion

This book is devoted and created for those of you who wish to change your own life and the life of others in a positive way. To create the change in your own life and the life of others. To hold onto your own power and increase your awareness of your own power by creating change yourself.

Perhaps even more importantly, this book is designed for the professional therapist who works with clients to assist them to come in touch with their own power. This book has techniques and procedures outlined and explained. It does, however, take into account that individual using these procedures has a very good grasp of concepts and a background in visualization techniques and/or

Neuro Linguistic Programming techniques. If the individual does not have this background they may choose to seek out a therapist who is an expert in that field.

For those of you who are already experts in the fields of Neuro Linguistic Programming, visualization techniques and therapy you will find extraordinary results with your clients.

Chapter Seven

Research

Body Contouring™: Hypnotic Alternatives to Surgery for Breast Augmentation and Liposuction

Abstract

This study incorporates a program combining group hypnosis, visualization, and subliminal tapes to enlarge women's breasts as well as to reduce the dimensions of the hips and thighs. The subjects increased an average of over 1.6 inches in the chest and over .75 inches in breast fullness. The subjects also decreased an average of nearly 2.5 inches in the upper hip, more than 1.75 inches in the lower hip, and an average of over 1.5 inches in the upper thigh.

Study

Society places a great deal of importance upon physical appearance. This is not a new phenomenon, but an extremely old one. As long people have had bodies, they have sought ways to make themselves more attractive or desirable to others. Individuals who were fortunate enough to possess a natural predisposition for the current

73

style often enjoyed much higher self-esteem than those left to painstakingly try and adapt to the current trend. Some trends have simply been hairstyles, or clothing fashions. Others have been much more, if not entirely, dependent upon body size, shape, and proportion. You could be considered quite fortunate indeed to have the ideal figure of the day, whatever that happened to be.

Individuals with high self-esteem do not always possess the "ideal" physical appearance. Certainly some do, and some don't, but somehow they do not seem to be particularly preoccupied by it. Individuals with lower self-esteem may feel that if their physical appearance were somehow different, that their life would improve. This may not be an entirely false concept. Certainly increased attractiveness can lead towards greater social acceptance and approachability. However, if the person does not possess a healthy self-esteem, then the overall results of a physical change could result in not only increased initial attraction and interactions, but also in increased rejection as a result of failure to live up to others expectations about the individual, based upon initial attraction. For this reason I would stress work on the self-esteem prior to, or at least concurrently with, any program designed to result in an outwardly visible change in physical appearance.

In the 1980's a great deal of cosmetic surgery moved from corrective surgery to elective surgery. The increase number of surgeries performed in breast augmentation and liposuction alone has been phenomenal. The old saying "You can't judge a book by it's cover" begins to have entirely new meaning.

Unfortunately these surgical techniques have many drawbacks. The virtually immediate result do not often allow the patient adequate time to prepare, or fully understand the far reaching, as well as limited, affect that these types of surgery can have upon their life. For example; a woman who elects to undergo surgery to increase her breast size from a A to a 34C may certainly experience the larger breast size. However, she may not achieve the increased self-esteem that she may actually be desiring as a result of the operation.

A second, and potentially life threatening aspect of these types of surgeries include; toxicity of implants; leakage; breakdown; increased development in other remaining cells; exposure to anesthesia; severity of the operation.

Other areas to address are the potential for scaring, loss of sensation, unnatural feel or appearance, recovery time, and cost.

Through the use of hypnosis many of the same results can be experienced. Granted, these results do take longer to manifest than a 4 hour surgery. However, they are 100% natural, no negative side effects, offer fantastic potential to improve the self-esteem, and can be administered at a fraction of the cost of surgery.

Rationale and Research Question

The earlier studies done on breast enlargement through hypnosis (Williams, 1974; Staib & Logan, 1977; Willard, 1977) appear to have been effective, though not widely utilized. The use of hypnosis for weight control has been widely acclaimed as successful. With the current trend towards health and women desiring larger breasts and smaller hips, we posed the following question:

The Research Question:

Can larger breasts and smaller hips, thighs, and buttocks be accomplished satisfactorily and simultaneously through the use of hypnosis?

Subjects:

Subjects in this study are women age 19-52. They were randomly chosen, and from a variety of educational, and socio-economic backgrounds.

Methods:

The subjects met one evening per week in a group to be measured and participate in group hypnosis. As in previous studies, this took place over a period of twelve weeks.

After initial group meetings to gather subjects the 20 subjects chosen met in groups of 4-12 one night a week for a period of 12 weeks. The subjects were then weighed and measured in a separate room, two at a time, by a researcher other than the hypnotherapist. In order to reduce any excessive external influences, expectations, or anxieties the subjects were not informed of the results of these measurements during the study. For the same reasons at no time did the hypnotherapist view the subjects breasts or results of the measurements.

Instrumentation and Measurement:

The device used for measurement was a 100CM cloth tape measure. The choice to use a metric rule was made in order to more closely monitor change, as well as to discourage subjects from easily recognizing dimensional changes from statistical familiarity.

Two different measurement techniques were used to quantify the breast growth portion of the study. Both techniques use measurements taken with the participant inhaled fully and exhaled fully in an attempt to eliminate breath position as a variable. The first technique measures the circumference of the chest cavity just below the breast, then across the nipples. The difference between these measurements represents the breast tissue itself. The second technique takes measurements from the bottom of the breast, to the nipple, then perpendicular to the clavicle. This measurement attempts to measure breast fullness and was taken individually for both the left and right breasts. The results are recorded in centimeters.

After completion of the measurements the subjects returned to the main treatment room and participated in a group hypnotic induction for both deepening the hypnotic state, and creating visualization techniques. These sessions initially lasted approximately 45 minutes.

On the fourth week the hypnotherapist began using a much shorter induction, based upon suggestions implanted in earlier sessions. The average session then lasted approximately 30 minutes.

The primary techniques used include age regression; assurances of individual control; visualization of changes; and age progression, visualizing attainment of their goal.

The subject of specific size, shape, or weight was never discussed during any interview, discussion of objectives, or during any hypnotic session. Suggestions for diet, exercise, rest, cell growth, cell nourishment, cell reduction and elimination were given. Suggestions that these processes would continue throughout every moment of the day and night were also given.

Results:

This Body Contouring research was conducted between October 1990 and January 1991. No attempt is made to judge the effectiveness of the study, the judgement is left to the reader. The results of the measurements were recorded in centimeters.

Another part of the body contouring study dealt with the hip and thigh areas. The two hip measurements were taken at the level of the sacrum/coccyx joint and the pubic mound.

The thigh measurement was taken where the leg meets the hip. Participant 0117 did not participate in the thigh portion of the study.

Discussion

The study started with twenty participants. Since many of the subjects were college students, the pressure of final exams and the winter holidays caused several participants to attend sporadically. Subjects who did not complete five or more sessions, of the total of twelve, were not included in the results. The subjects who did not complete five sessions are 0103, 0106, 0107, 0108, 0109, 0110, 0116 and 0119.

Although it was not specifically addressed, weight was recorded on a weekly basis for all participants. The average weight variance for all subjects was 5.09 pounds.

One subject had a hysterectomy and showed the least breast growth of the group. It may be speculated that the capability of the body to produce the necessary hormones may have been greatly reduced. However, the subject reported great satisfaction with the results attained, supporting the validity of good self-esteem.

One subject (who did not complete the study) reported a slight loss in breast size after a six-month follow-up. It is mentioned here in order to note that there were no suggestions given for maintenance of size or increase until after the 8th week. This subject had increased over 4" in her breasts (over 2 cup sizes) in 5 weeks. At that point she discontinued the study, prior to receiving any suggestions for maintenance.

Other physical changes reported by subjects included loss or reduction of stretch marks, cellulite, wrinkles, and scars. There were also claims of hair regrowth on the scalp. These are reports made by the subjects, and were not specifically addressed or documented in this study.

The psychological changes reported by subjects included better overall feelings about themselves, their life, their attitude, their sleep, and increased energy levels.

Conclusion

To summarize, the participants gained an average of over 1.6 inches in the chest and over .75 inches in breast fullness. The participants also lost an average of nearly 2.5 inches in the upper hip and over 1.75 inches in the lower hip. The participants also lost an average of over 1.5 inches in the upper thigh.

The results of this study would appear to indicate that hypnosis is indeed a very viable and effective alternative to plastic surgery, producing similar, if not identical results. Hypnosis allows the subject to play a much more involved role in their own transformation. This once again adds to the subject's own self-esteem and confidence.

Suggestions for Future Research

Some researchers may chose to address the possibility of achieving faster results with either longer sessions, or through the use of multiple sessions per week. Other promising areas for research would appear to be in the areas of stretch marks, cellulite, wrinkle, and scar reduction, as well as hair restoration.

Breast measurement 1 results (table 1):

Subject	Inhaled					Exhaled				
Number	Min	Max	Var	SDev	d	Min	Max	Var	SDev	d
0101	9.9	13.6	1.25	1.12	3.7	10.1	14.7	1.53	1.24	4.6
0102	9.3	11.9	0.59	0.77	2.6	8.2	12.2	1.99	1.41	4.0
0104	11.0	17.2	4.00	2.00	6.2	11.3	18.5	4.34	2.08	7.2
0105	7.0	10.7	1.33	1.15	3.7	7.0	10.3	1.45	1.21	3.3
0111	8.9	11.5	1.05	1.02	2.6	8.5	11.3	1.27	1.13	2.8
0112	7.4	13.1	3.67	1.91	5.7	7.5	12.0	2.15	1.46	4.5
0113	6.5	9.6	1.02	1.01	3.1	7.4	9.5	0.51	0.71	2.1
0114	10.0	15.6	3.19	1.79	5.6	9.8	14.3	2.09	1.45	4.5
0115	5.9	12.6	3.98	1.99	6.7	7.0	13.0	2.97	1.73	6.0
0117	11.7	15.2	1.24	1.11	3.5	12.0	14.4	0.63	0.79	2.4
0120	8.4	12.1	1.73	1.31	3.7	8.3	12.2	2.27	1.51	3.9
ave					4.28					4.12
					1.69"					1.62"

Breast measurement 2 results (table 2):

Subject Number		Min	Max	Var	SDev	d	Min	Max	Var	SDev	d
			Inhaled					**Exhaled**			
0101	R	26.5	27.6	0.14	0.38	1.1	26.0	27.6	0.23	0.47	1.6
	L	25.6	27.5	0.18	0.43	1.9	25.5	27.5	0.25	0.49	2.0
0102	R	29.5	31.7	0.62	0.78	2.2	29.5	31.7	0.62	0.78	2.2
	L	30.0	32.5	0.48	0.69	2.5	30.0	32.5	0.48	0.69	2.5
0104	R	34.0	36.5	0.63	0.79	2.5	34.0	36.5	0.63	0.79	2.5
	L	33.0	35.5	0.55	0.74	2.5	33.0	35.5	0.55	0.74	2.5
0105	R	29.0	31.0	0.63	0.79	2.0	29.0	31.0	0.63	0.79	2.5
	L	26.0	27.5	0.28	0.53	1.5	26.0	27.5	0.28	0.53	1.5
0111	R	31.5	33.0	0.26	0.51	1.5	31.5	33.0	0.26	0.51	1.5
	L	30.5	32.7	0.59	0.77	2.2	30.5	32.7	0.59	0.77	2.2
0112	R	27.0	32.0	2.96	1.72	5.0	26.8	32.0	3.10	1.76	5.2
	L	27.0	31.7	3.12	1.77	4.7	26.8	31.7	3.33	1.82	4.9
0113	R	28.0	29.0	0.17	0.41	1.0	27.8	29.0	0.19	0.44	1.2
	L	28.0	29.0	0.12	0.34	1.0	27.9	29.0	0.13	0.36	1.1
0114	R	29.0	30.0	0.24	0.49	1.0	29.0	30.0	0.20	0.45	1.0
	L	29.0	30.0	0.18	0.43	1.0	28.8	30.0	0.20	0.45	1.2
0115	R	27.0	29.0	0.37	0.61	2.0	27.0	29.0	0.34	0.61	2.0
	L	26.0	28.5	0.44	0.67	2.5	26.0	28.5	0.44	0.67	2.5
0117	R	30.8	31.8	0.11	0.33	1.0	30.8	31.8	0.11	0.33	1.0
	L	30.2	31.8	0.24	0.49	1.6	30.2	31.8	0.24	0.49	1.6
0120	R	22.8	25.0	0.48	0.69	2.2	22.8	25.0	0.48	0.69	2.2
	L	22.8	25.0	0.52	0.72	2.2	22.8	25.0	0.52	0.72	2.2
ave	R				1.95					2.04	
					0.77"					0.80"	
	L				2.15					2.20	
					0.85"					0.87"	

Hip measurement results (table 3):

Subject	Hip 1					Hip 2				
Number	Min	Max	Var	SDev	d	Min	Max	Var	SDev	d
0101	87.0	94.0	3.54	1.88	7.0	96.1	99.5	1.36	1.16	3.4
0102	85.4	93.5	5.62	2.37	8.1	94.0	98.0	1.61	1.27	4.0
0104	96.4	100.0	1.85	1.36	3.6	104.0	106.3	0.58	0.76	2.3
0105	87.9	92.0	2.01	1.42	4.1	93.0	97.9	3.40	1.84	4.9
0111	100.1	104.0	1.66	1.28	3.9	105.7	107.8	0.67	0.82	2.1
0112	82.5	94.0	15.56	3.94	11.5	89.9	95.5	3.81	1.95	5.6
0113	96.0	99.0	1.24	1.11	3.0	97.8	100.7	1.15	1.07	2.9
0114	96.1	101.5	2.91	1.70	5.4	101.6	104.0	0.69	0.83	2.4
0115	79.8	88.7	6.99	2.64	8.9	80.5	91.0	14.45	3.80	10.5
0117	86.5	94.9	7.71	2.77	8.4	90.6	99.0	6.27	2.50	8.4
0120	80.4	85.0	2.66	1.63	4.6	87.4	90.5	1.57	1.25	3.1
ave				6.23					4.51	
				2.45"					1.78"	

Thigh measurement results (table 4):

Subject Number		Min	Max	Var	SDev	d
0101	R	56.5	65.0	5.12	2.26	8.5
	L	58.2	65.0	3.86	1.96	6.8
0102	R	57.5	60.0	0.41	0.64	2.5
	L	58.0	60.7	0.69	0.83	2.7
0104	R	60.6	67.7	4.99	2.23	7.1
	L	61.8	67.0	2.67	1.63	5.2
0105	R	54.3	60.0	4.84	2.20	5.7
	L	53.6	60.0	6.58	2.56	6.4
0111	R	63.7	64.5	0.07	0.27	0.8
	L	64.3	66.0	0.39	0.62	1.7
0112	R	52.0	56.0	1.99	1.41	4.0
	L	52.0	57.0	3.23	1.79	5.0
0113	R	56.8	62.0	4.29	2.07	5.2
	L	59.0	67.3	6.12	2.47	7.7
0114	R	60.0	66.3	5.20	2.28	6.3
	L	61.0	66.8	4.70	2.17	5.8
0120	R	49.0	53.2	1.95	1.39	4.2
	L	50.0	52.5	0.76	0.87	2.5
ave	R					4.03
						1.59"
	L					3.98
						1.57"

Thigh 1

Chapter Eight

Results

The Body Contouring Programme^{TM} was initially developed as a response to the desire of women to increase breast size. Review of the research findings from the original study covered in Chapter 7 will reveal that those results were realized. However, in the discussion section of the original research you will also find that many other physical changes were experienced as well. Women in the study reported a reduction in size of the thighs, hips, buttocks, abdomen and other very specific spot reductions. Cellulite reduction or apparent elimination was also reported by the participants in the study. As one woman described it, "It was as though someone had taken an clothes iron and put it on the back of my thighs and just ironed everything out nice and smooth." Others reported reduction or elimination of wrinkling, scars and stretch marks. Increased suppleness and overall skin tonicity was significantly observable. Other reported results included thickening of hair and an overall "youthing" process.

In addition the participants in the original study reported an overall toning of the body. Participants of the research program also reported a sense of increased levels of energy, vitality and sensuality.

There has been an almost universal improvement in sensuality and sexuality among clients. Many clients report improved or renewed relationships. Others started new relationships and/or careers. These changes are typically the result of improving the self-concept and self-esteem of the individual. This has been very positive in all cases.

The typical *Body Contouring Programme*^{TM} client has been female. That is virtually the only thing that all the clients have had in common. However, the same techniques that have been successfully implemented with female clients can be modified to work with male clients. Recently we have been working in the area of hair restoration. We are developing some scripts at the time of this writing. The clients and therapists that we have worked with at this time are reporting positive results.

The other similarities between clients are that they are all different. The reasons that women have cited for wanting change in their physical appearance vary from individual to individual. Their background is varied from individual to individual.

Our original experience with *The Body Contouring Programme*^{TM} was in Southern California. The majority of the women who inquired into the program desired larger breasts. However, there were also a significant number of women who desired breast reductions.

When we conducted seminars in different cultures we found that the societal image of what was desirable varied. This of course changed the desires and interests of the participants in the program. In all cases participants have reported satisfactorily on their results or desired outcomes.

We hasten to point out that during our research, only visualization and specific languaging techniques were utilized to achieve the results detailed in Chapter Seven. There were no specific suggestions given for diet or exercise plans. These were intentionally avoided during the study. Subsequently, throughout our research and with other clients, we have found that the addition of specific exercise and/or dietary suggestion have indeed effected change even more rapidly.

How do these physical changes come about?

The individual creates a very specific, very intense image of themselves. An image of the way they would choose to be. It is your responsibility or opportunity as a therapist to create an intense, compelling, fully associated experience for the individual.

We're not going to suggest that change happens instantaneously, overnight or even within a few days or weeks. Individual's results vary just as people vary. The amount of time required to fully attain the desired outcome depends upon the amount of change desired.

However, one apparent underlying factor for success in the program is the frequency or repetition of exposure to the material. We have had clients who were seen on a weekly basis. Certainly from the first week to the second week there were measurable, visually apparent changes. In many cases the clients themselves were very aware and thrilled with the changes. There have also been clients for whom it took four or five weeks to really notice change. That's not to say there were not measurable changes, indeed, there were. Their charts definitely depicted their progress. In some of these instances it had taken the client over a month to realize and accept the changes in themselves.

We learned from the apparent unwillingness of these clients to accept positive changes in themselves and we stress the importance of a thorough intake and utilization of Time Line Therapy™ to assist in removing limiting thoughts and beliefs. Assisting the client in creating and maintaining a positive attitude is of tremendous value to assure rapid success in this program.

Measuring and Monitoring

Our experience has been to measure the client thoroughly with the 12 different measurements we utilized in the breast enlargement study contained earlier in chapter 7. We had participants measured weekly for the duration of the study.

We have found that the client seems to feel a greater amount of professional concern when measured on a weekly basis. There also seems to be a strong desire on the part of the client to perform and participate in increasing or decreasing their physical shape when measured weekly. It is as though it becomes a "team" effort. This lead to a high level of subject motivation and involvement.

During the study we kept these actual measurements from the clients for the duration of the study. We did however let them know that their measurements were being charted. In future sessions we found when the clients had not been measured on a weekly basis, their performance was not as rapid as it had been when measured on a weekly basis.

Allow us once again to point out that measuring clients is something we had chosen to have done by doctors other than ourselves. However you may choose to do that in you own office. You might chose to use a nurse or another professional. It has consistently been our practice to refrain from having ever seen any of our clients disrobe in any manner. We have chosen to do this in order to keep professional distance there as well as to avoid potential for negative media portrayal.

The actual results of the initial study are addressed in chapter 7. Since that time numerous changes have occurred. Most exciting for us perhaps is the increased self-concept and self-esteem of the individual. The most exciting aspect of *The Body Contouring Programme*™ for participants varies from individual to individual (as well it should).

III

Processes Involved in

The Body Contouring Programme™

Chapter Nine

Techniques

We have been particularly cautious in developing *The Body Contouring Programme*^{TM} in order to avoid the obvious opportunities for the media to exploit the practice and results. There has certainly been some light-hearted attention already given to similar, less researched practices. The procedures and techniques which are being utilized within *The Body Contouring Programme*^{TM} result in the greatest, most consistent and all-encompassing results of any program currently taking place.

In addition to our media concerns the question of the motivation of therapist has on occasion been in question. In an attempt to reduce the possibility for negative press we have opted to use a doctor other than ourselves to do all measuring of the client during therapy.

Through research, study, experience and observation we have developed *The Body Contouring Programme*^{TM}. The basic tool in *The Body Contouring Programme*^{TM} may at first appear to be visualization. Certainly visualization is a large part of the program. However visualization is actually more a form of delivery of several components.

The exposure to different techniques and theories and the eclectic combination of those techniques and theories that have lead to the unequaled results of this program. The major techniques utilized in *The Body Contouring Programme*™ include aspects of Hypnosis, Neuro Linguistic Programming and Time Line Therapy™. Even with all of our background and training the outcome of this program are the result of the client's implementation of the techniques. Integral to the success of this program is the client's willingness to review and reassess his or her beliefs.

We strongly encourage familiarization with the techniques taught in Time Line Therapy™ (chapter 5). We have found these techniques to be some of the most effective in modifying limiting decisions and beliefs. These techniques are virtually essential to prepare the client for the changes that will be taking place. It is for that reason certification as a *Body Contouring Programme*™ Practitioner requires certification as a Time Line Therapy™ Practitioner.

Your clients will actually experiencing themselves in their perceived state of perfection; the size, shape, and proportion of their body. When they fully associate into that state, their body, the neurology within their body actually has that experience. The unconscious mind accepts this experience as real. When fully congruent the individual accepts this new belief. Your client sees, feels, and experiences this new physical state. This in turn creates a state of dissidence within the mind. It is one of the responsibilities of the unconscious mind to allow the body to shift into this new shape. Your body must come into alignment with these newly held beliefs. The body you or your client has outwardly displays the physical appearance based upon the internal perception held of their self.

Your mind is powerful, perhaps the greatest aspect of creating your health. Creating and maintaining your physical body, your energy levels, allowing blood flow to increase and decrease. Monitoring your metabolic and cardio-vascular rates to increase and decrease. These are all controlled by an aspect of your unconscious mind.

The Body Contouring Programme^{TM} begins by first completing a very thorough intake with the client. This includes becoming aware of what their outcome is, what their past has been, their up-bringing, their life to this point and what their goals and aspirations are.

If you're competent in your ability to evaluate a client you will probably require two hours to complete the intake phase. Important in this intake is the ability to recognize the causes of their limiting decisions or beliefs. Ideally the point in time in which the decisions were made if the client is consciously aware of them. If they are not consciously aware of the decision, or if it is not prior to age 15 then the use of Time Line Therapy^{TM} becomes invaluable.

We have found through our own practice and consulting with colleagues, if you do not do at least an hour and a half or more personal history on the client, then you are certainly overlooking some possibilities. We certainly feel that anything less is not doing a thorough intake and assessment into the client's reasoning and desire for change.

Neuro Linguistic Programming provides us with techniques for reprogramming your unconscious mind to allow you to create your new outcome. The opportunity to fully experience your new outcome. To instruct the cells to realign, reshape and reform in the manner appropriate to allow the desired changes to manifest. To experience outward physical changes... real, positive, physical change.

Understanding the client's full outcome and model of the world allows the competent therapist to assist the client in realizing rapid and effective changes. Once again calling attention to the client's own choice.

What is the underlying motivation for these changes?

Do they come in because their husband or their boyfriend thought they should have breast implants or larger breasts? Are your clients' just doing this just for themselves? It's important to assist them in realizing their true motivation for desiring a change. To allow yourself as the therapist to become the mirror for the client to assist them becoming more in touch with the reasoning, the beliefs and acknowledging their own power of decisions. To do this we utilize the detailed personal history.

As pointed out earlier, the primary reasons for change are poor self-concept or self-esteem issues. Even though this is *The Body Contouring Programme*^{TM}, the ultimate goal is mental, emotional and spiritual alignment for your client. When your client has full congruency their whole life will change. This includes the outward physical manifestations. We have found that as the client feels happier, healthier, stronger and more independent the changes occur even more rapidly.

Most of our clients are not aware consciously of which point in time they made a decision or how it came about. This is however a potentially crucial aspect of discovery. This sets the groundwork or "frame" to demonstrate their choice and their power. This is the opportunity to acknowledge the power and choice that the individual has. To recognize how much control that they do and have had in their life. This is very important to build upon. The concept that the individual has a choice. They made a choice once and have lived with it. Now they simply change their mind. Make a new choice. A conscious choice. A mature responsible choice, rather than one made as a response to a situation or others' beliefs.

If a client is not aware of when they made a decision as to their physical appearance then we utilize Time Line Therapy™. In many ways this might be considered a process of regression. However it is the fastest and "cleanest" way to assist them in getting in touch with the point in time where they made their limiting decisions or beliefs.

Having addressed the limiting decisions or beliefs it is every bit as important as to acknowledge the bases of their decisions now. Why have they come to you? Could it be simply for body contouring, breast enlargement, thigh reduction or spot reductions?

Another reason for the extended intake session is to administer several suggestibility tests to the client. Most if not all of these tests are given without their necessary awareness. These suggestibility tests are designed to assist the therapist in calibrating to the client and establishing an even deeper state of rapport. This is essential before we begin to move on to the first formal session of visualization.

Typical Program

In addition to the initial intake we strongly recommend that the client receive a physical performed by a medical doctor. This establishes several things. First, it establishes the client as a healthy individual. Second, it creates a more professional program. Third, it establishes a working relationship with physicians. This third situation can lead to much greater success down the road as the physician observes the changes that have taken place. It may be advisable for you as a therapist to locate a physician in your area to work with. You would certainly desire a physician who is well informed about the scope and intentions of *The Body Contouring Programme*^{TM}. This will assist both the client and the therapist in receiving maximum support for their efforts.

Upon completion of a very in depth personal history and establishment of rapport we introduce the client to a very deep trance. It's typically done with a very long induction to induce a very, very deep state of relaxation and focused attention on the part of the client.

After having compiled a complete and very thorough personal history on the individual, having decided what the actual cause or limiting belief that the individual believes is possible for size and shape of the body, you would begin by introducing them into a very relaxed state and perhaps using regression techniques early on.

Take the client back to the time of first awareness of the body. As the client becomes aware of his or her body, increase and heighten that awareness, bringing attention to feelings that were there or beliefs that were held. Was there uncertainty of a situation? Utilize the opportunity to integrate the maturity and wisdom of the person they are now. Speak with the child, who was uncertain and unaware of what was going on, and answer the question that perhaps even the child didn't know to ask, always surround it with a great deal of love and respect.

Consider doing this as a very nurturing, loving process. Facilitate the client in creating greater security, greater rapport, deeper concentration and focused awareness. Encourage a more intimate awareness of the body. Remind the client of that awareness with each breath and the movement of the body with each breath. At a point make reference to the pulsing of their heart and tie into blood flow.

Let the client become aware of not only the blood's responsibility of delivering oxygen and nutrients to all the cells of the body but also aware of the responsibility and capability of the blood to remove the excesses, in all parts of the body, and that through a normal process of elimination, all things leave the body.

And then draw attention to growth in the body, of the replacement, frequency in which cells are replaced. You know such things as we receive a new stomach lining every 5 days, or a new skin every 30 days as per Deepak Chopra's book, *Quantum Healing*, you may choose to get even more examples of that based on your own experience, reference, knowledge, include much of that into the pre-talk, pre-framing that's to take place as well as including it now in the body of the visualization or imagery work that you're doing. Allow the cells that are in another part of their body, such as their buttocks, their thighs, their abdomen, let it decrease in size there and increase in their breasts, and that any of those techniques would be fine, they simply allow it now. Give these suggestions with an authoritarian approach.

At this point, depending upon the client's needs or desires, suggestions to allow reduction to take place in parts of the body may be appropriate.

Often we will record the session on tape and give this to the client. Making the suggestion that they listen to the tape at least five times within the next week. Preferably daily or twice daily. The results have shown that the greater frequency that the client uses the tape, the greater the speed and amount of change that takes place.

We are aware of therapists who do not record their sessions. They do not use tapes. Some may use generic tapes developed specifically for this initially. There are different approaches and certainly different techniques.

We have found through our experiences that the greatest results have been achieved when doing a live tape and giving a copy of that to the client. This has provided both a greater sense of comfort on the part of the client as well as a greater amount of personal attention, commitment and bond between the therapist and the client.

This bond or cooperative spirit also seems to encourage the client to perform even more rapidly, to perform well for the therapist, thereby making the therapist an even a greater success. After all, that is what we're after, making both the client and the therapist a success.

After the initial visit and intake the client then begins a 10 week program. This program may begin on the first session. The initial session consists of a very specific, very deep, initial induction and visualization process. At this time specific post-hypnotic suggestions are installed. At the end of this session a cassette tape of the induction is provided for them. The instructions are to listen to the tape at least five times during the following week (preferably twice daily). The client is also given a daily journal to keep for the duration of the program.

It is recommended that the client be given a tape to listen to a minimum of five times the first week. However, the greater the frequency of repetition of use of the tape the greater the involvement of the client in the visualization process. Research has shown that the more frequently the client listens to the tapes the faster they assimilate the information and the sooner they allow integration of mind and body to take place. In deed the results have shown statistically that the women who listened to their tapes a minimum of twice a day have far and away the fastest and greatest results.

The second session is shorter. Approximately one hour in length. Again, the client is given a new cassette tape (much shorter in length). After the second session the client follows up with a weekly session for the next nine weeks creating a ten week program in total.

Another purpose for the detailed personal history is to become aware of any additional areas of therapy that might be warranted to assist the client in realizing their total outcome. This provides the therapist with a more accurate client profile. If the therapist is highly skilled or trained in NLP they will also be aware of the client's lead and primary representational systems.

After the initial session, weekly follow-ups for the next 8 to 10 weeks are recommended, subsequent sessions would recommend, in my experiences a one hour follow-up the end of week one and to have much more intake experience, participation with the client and then culminating with a new tape being generated on a shorter duration, perhaps only 15 or 20 minutes, something that can be easily used. After having listened to the first tape, the deep induction, and having put a subliminal suggestion, a post hypnotic suggestion in an easy client achieve the state of visualization readily and easily.

After the second session I continue to see clients on a weekly basis, perhaps only a 30 minute session, perhaps longer if you'd care to have more feedback or if you're doing additional therapy with the client, in which case you may choose to use an hour or more. And at which point in time by the third visit, a generic tape would seem to be appropriate and quite usable if you would choose to go this route.

Continuing in this vein often by the fifth week, the client will have had 4 tapes to listen to and they have typically find one which they would prefer over the others or tend to listen to more frequently than the others.

At which point we may discuss that and even make a particularly special tape for the client. Perhaps looking at a bit more time for that, perhaps making the tape at another time altogether without the client being present. That's up to the therapist's own schedule, style, techniques. Refrain from any reference to maintenance of breast growth or thigh reduction or of any physical changes until the 7th week.

The first 6 weeks have been devoted to developing the physical body, redefining that image and holding it, specifically, in it's increasing the growth and size of the breasts or decreasing the size of the thighs, hips, buttocks or abdomen or skin tonicity. The first 6 weeks are all geared towards change. Again, any suggestion regarding maintenance is reserved for the 7th session.

In the 7th week, begin to introduce the concept of maintenance and permanence with this new size and shape. Indeed, in the 8th session, particularly if that's a final session, heavily emphasis future pacing, maintenance and permanence.

Conclusion

Some suggestions for scripts are included later in this text in Chapter Eleven, as well as being available in a series of auditory tapes from *The Body Contouring Programme*™. In addition to these audio tapes there are seminars and trainings being conducted throughout the world.

Information on *The Body Contouring Programme*™ seminars and trainings, or information on certified practitioners of *The Body Contouring Programme*™ are available by contacting the International Association of *Body Contouring Programme*™ Practitioners.

Chapter Ten

Areas of Importance

In many books there is one chapter which really stands out in the reader's mind. The chapter that ties it all together. The chapter that sums it up. If you are the type of person who just wants the basic considerations. If you don't care about the how and why. If being aware of the history, research and development of a program bores you... this is your chapter.

If you have studied the text so far (you know who you are) much of this may seem redundant to you. However, remember... redundancy increases accuracy. After all, you have bought or borrowed this book. You have invested your time in reading it. Now how about actually utilizing it for something more than conversation.

We encourage you to use these successful techniques in your own life and practice. In our experience they always work. Let us repeat that. The techniques, when applied as we have described and use ourselves, always work.

So if you have been looking for a "cheat sheet", this chapter is the answer.

Perhaps the most important consideration before you see even your first client is "Can my client achieve their outcome?". If you can undeniably say yes to this question then please continue. If you have any doubts or limiting beliefs what so ever, please refer the client out. Remember the client will absolutely realize the therapist's expectations.

Motivation of the Client

Why is the client there? What is their expressed motivation? What do they hope to accomplish in these sessions? Have they tried before? If so, what were the results. Why haven't they been able to accomplish the changes on their own? Do they have a secondary gain? What type of investment do they have in accomplishing their desired change? Are they congruent with their answers?

It has been my experience and belief, as well as others, that individuals are totally responsible for their own changes taking place. In fact one of the basic premises of NLP is that "An individual has all of the resources necessary to change.". Another major premise is that "An individual is utilizing the best options that they have available at a given time." If we fully accept these two premises then we can proceed to assist an individual in transforming their own life. Part of assisting an individual in transforming their life is by establishing fully in their own mind that they are the cause of all (or at least the majority) of things in their life.

There is a widely held belief that we are either at cause or at effect in our lives. That is to say we either cause things to happen in our lives, or we are experiencing what is the result of things happening to us.

A simple equation of this is:

$$C > E$$

Cause   Effect

Is the individual the cause of the things going on in their life, or is their life the result of external influences? Are they making conscious decisions in their life, or are the decisions being made for them?

It may sound a bit philosophical, however the answer is no. No, the person is not making fully conscious decision in their life. No, as much as they might like to think they are, others are not totally responsible for the events and experiences in another person's life.

Enter here the concept of choice. There are several theories on how much choice we actually have. Some individuals believe that we have absolute choice over everything that happens in our lives. We have a choice where we live, if and who we marry, if and where we work and even the time of our birth and family we were born into. We have a choice whether to remain in a situation or to move on.

On the other end of this perhaps continuum is we have little or no choice, the concept of fate. The belief that a person is pre-destined to experience all of the things that happen in their life. The most extreme cases of this believe that the individual is powerless to effect any change in their life. The belief that they are but a pawn in the larger game of life.

One could certainly argue that having the belief that they are powerless in their life is indeed a choice. One could also argue that an individual was pre-destined to have more personal power in their life. In either case, it is the acknowledgement of another individual's beliefs that is important. It is also important to point out that in acknowledging another individual's beliefs you do not have to agree with them or accept them as your own.

In order to be successful in this program you must reach agreement with yourself or your client as to how this program will effect the individual. It is essential in the very beginning of the program that you hold and exercise the belief that the individual is the cause of at least the majority, if not all of the things in their life.

In the case of the individual that defaults to a higher power, you need simply point out that they have been given the opportunity for the experience. The tools are being made available for their use. Opportunity has knocked, will they answer the door?

What specific changes does the client hope to make? Keep in mind that *The Body Contouring Programme*^{TM} was developed primarily to work with the self-concept. Certainly physical changes, often dramatic, will occur as the program is implemented. It is however beneficial, if not absolutely mandatory, to have a clear understanding as to the desired outcome of the program. By discussing in-depth the desired outcome you begin to establish a deeper rapport and understanding of the client. As you undergo this process you will often discover hidden or underlying reasons for the desired changes. Through the effective use of probing questions and follow-up you may discover a secondary gain that the individual has for either succeeding or failing with the program. In the event that this occurs you may want to use a reframe or integration technique to modify the client's previously held belief.

Well seasoned therapists or NLP practitioners may perform the intervention as part of the intake session. Individuals beginning to work in this field may either want to suggest additional therapy prior to starting the program, or refer the client out.

As part of the initial discussion and intake it is important to establish the history of the individual. What types of therapies or programs have they been exposed to or involved with? Establish what, if anything, was successful or beneficial about the program. Determine what didn't work. Ask for their opinion as to why it didn't work. They know why it didn't work. If they offer the answer that they "don't know", ask them again. This is very important. I can save both you and your client a great deal of time. Be persistent! If everything they ever tried worked they would not be in front of you now.

I made reference to the client being in front of you. You may choose to gain a few answers over the telephone or through a written questionnaire. In fact the use of an extensive questionnaire can often be an invaluable tool. It can either be filled out by the individual or by an interviewer or screener at the time the initial appointment is made. However it is imperative that you have as much information as possible available as you begin the program. It allows you to utilize the nonverbal channels as well as provide immediate feedback and investigation into matters that might otherwise be overlooked or omitted.

After all of these other areas have been discussed (or concurrently, depending upon your interviewing style) it is very important to discuss commitment. While many, if not all of your clients are motivated initially, an 8 - 10 week program can become quite long.

Be aware that you may become not only the client's therapist, but quite possibly their coach and motivator.

Remember, all things being equal (which is virtually impossible), the most significant variable in the speed and success of *The Body Contouring Programme*^{TM} is consistency and frequency. The client who allows him or herself a quiet, uninterrupted half-hour two or more times a day consistently will statistically achieve the fastest and most significant results.

Financial considerations are often a concern. The experience reported in this program is comparable to most others. If the therapy is not paid in full at the onset of the program then the potential for negative reinforcement exists. This certainly does not benefit the client. The issue surrounding guarantees is similar. If a person requires a money-back guarantee they are almost certainly asking for permission to fail. Each therapist must address these issues on a personal basis, just as value of the program to the client in relation to the therapist's time.

At the time of this writing in 1993 it was not uncommon to have a fee of $300.00 per hour and up for an experienced NLP practitioner. Therefore an 8-week, 10-hour program would be pried accordingly. The overall benefit of *The Body Contouring Programme*^{TM} includes mental, emotional as well as the non-invasive physical aspects for the individual. Coupled with the rapidness of the overall change the value of the program has been quite well received.

After a thorough discussion of each of these program components and concepts check the individual for congruency of understanding and acceptance of the principles to be utilized. If you discover any resistance or incongruence to exist make sure and address it in this initial session. If it can be resolved, great. If it cannot, or the individual is primarily interested in changing to please someone other than him or herself you may choose to suggest other therapy with either yourself or another therapist before continuing with the program.

Accepting an individual who is only partially willing or uncertain about any aspect of change or what is required of them in the program introduces an unnecessary opportunity for a less than optimal experience for both the client and the therapist.

Performing the Intake

Have you scheduled enough time to perform an in-depth intake? Did you accomplish unconscious rapport? Are you aware of the client's lead and primary representational systems? Is the client normal or reverse organized? Has the client responded favorably to suggestibility tests? Do you clearly identify the components and different levels of compliance? Have you discussed who is responsible and in control?

In my experience, and that of several of my colleagues, a three-hour intake session seems to be optimal. I have certainly been asked; "What do you do for three hours?" by therapists as well as clients. The clients are easy. You simply explain that it takes that long to extract all of the information necessary to develop an effective personal program for the individual.

Therapists on the other hand can be quite resistive to this approach. Unfortunately many therapists are still locked into the concept and practice of the 50-minute therapy hour. The techniques and interventions employed in *The Body Contouring Programme*™ as well as in other advanced techniques of NLP and Time Line Therapy™ can actually take very few minutes. The results of these techniques and interventions can be extremely beneficial. Often the results can lead to significant lifestyle changes. The execution and implementation of these techniques relies upon the thorough and efficient gathering of information.

The initial three-hour intake session allows the therapist the opportunity to gather information at an apparently more relaxed pace. The client is often less concerned with providing brief answers. The awareness of adequate time to discuss issues is important. It allows for a more relaxed intake.

The skilled therapist is utilizing virtually every word or nonverbal response given by the client during this initial intake session. Determination as to which representational system (visual, auditory or kinesthetic) is being used as the lead system. Determination as to whether the lead system is the same as the primary representational system. Attention to the modal operators used is important.

Upon making initial determinations it is important to test for accuracy. Is the client normal or reverse organized? As you determine validity of your observations you can begin checking for strategies or programs that are currently being utilized.

During this process you may chose to check for unconscious rapport through the use of language, mirroring or matching of physical behavior. As you establish unconscious rapport begin to lead or modify the behavior. Having accomplished this, begin to introduce suggestibility tests.

You may choose to use covert suggestibility tests at first. As you perceive compliance and receive positive feedback you may chose to explain some of the tests you have used and the client's response. This is very important. Once the client has responded favorably to one or more suggestibility tests point them out. They may be as simple as a request for the client to reposition their hands or to take a deep breath.

Anything that presupposes trance induces trance. Maintain a positive, confident, in control attitude at all times. Your client will manifest the beliefs that you hold about them. If you have any doubts about your ability to assist a client in achieving positive results from sessions with you refer them elsewhere.

It is important to discuss the different level of compliance or trance. Explain the varying aspects or characteristics of these states. You may compare them to the suggestibility tests. Explain the differences between up-time and down-time trances. Discuss the naturally occurring states, as well as the frequency or cycles in which they occur. It is important to explain briefly how the actual process of focused attention works. Certainly an important component of this discussion is the process of termination or conclusion of the trance state. Explain what happens if the therapist stops talking in the middle of a session or a tape stops. Make it very clear to the client that they are always in control.

Control is a major concern. The client needs to be aware that all hypnosis is self-hypnosis. That the therapist is only a tour guide. A highly skilled and highly trained tour guide. However the individual is doing all of the work. The therapist in this respect is like a coach. The client performs mental workouts several times throughout the week and reports back with the results. The therapist then proceeds to modify or reinforce the program to assist the individual in attaining their outcome or goal. The most important aspect of this program is personal empowerment and improved self-concept. The client is always responsible for their achievements.

Sessions

Is the client following through on their commitment? Do they keep their appointments? Are you, as a therapist, remaining optimistic and encouraging?

This is an extremely effective program. The major key to success is commitment, execution and follow through. I cannot emphasize enough the importance of a daily routine, an almost ritualistic use of the program. The greater the consistency and use of the program the greater and faster the results.

The weekly sessions with the therapist are designed for feedback and modification of the program if necessary. They are also used to address individual issues that may be dealt with concurrently with *The Body Contouring Programme*^{TM}. In addition these sessions act as reinforcement session. An opportunity to share successes and/or to voice concerns. The weekly sessions provide the continued support and commitment for the client on behalf of the therapist.

If a client begins to miss or consistently reschedule appointments it may be a strong indication of lack of commitment. If this is the case then the success of the program may be minimized. To avoid this potential situation or outcome stress the importance of the commitment of both the therapist and the client. Set a definite appointment schedule and maintain it whenever possible.

As the therapist it is your responsibility and obligation to remain positive and optimistic. Remember, you believed that your client can obtain the goals that you have agreed upon or you would not have accepted them as a client.

Tapes

How often do they listen to their tapes? Are you using personally created tapes or pre-recorded ones? How many different tapes do you provide your client? Are all representational systems present in the tapes? Are you addressing the areas of interest of the client? Does the client enjoy the tapes? What are the client's favorite parts of the tapes? Does the client remember the tapes?

The greater the frequency that the client listens to the tapes seems to have a direct correlation to the speed and amount of changes that takes place. For optimum results I recommend the client listen to the tapes three times a day. Typically first thing in the morning, again at mid-day or afternoon and finally as they go to sleep at night. It is important that the client listen to the tapes at a time when they are free from other distractions or interruptions.

When I first began developing *The Body Contouring Programme*^{TM} I created new tapes for each client live at each session. Over the years I have developed and refined a series of six audio cassettes that I now use exclusively. I will typically see a client in the office and use a spontaneous induction with specific suggestions relating to the items discussed during that day's session. However it is very seldom that I will record these sessions. Upon special request or need I will create specific tapes for a client.

The tapes that I create are approximately 20 minutes in length. They have a *wake-up* side for morning and daytime use and a *sleep* side for regenerative nighttime use. I utilize clinically developed and tested progressive relaxation background music. The music is important to first of all integrate both the right and left hemispheres of the brain. Secondly, the specific music that I use matches sound and vibration with the individual endocrine glands or chakra systems. Thirdly, it establishes an auditory anchor.

The first tape in my series is a very slow, deep induction, general use tape. It does contain agreement frames and indirect as well as direct suggestions. The tape is used as an anchor, which is accessed and built upon with subsequent tapes. The four tapes that make up the body of the tape series are complexly simply visualizations. The tapes each address different areas of personal development. The sixth tape contains suggestions about maintenance and future pacing.

Through the specific design of these tapes a single 20-minute tape allows the client the restorative value of a 90-minute nap. After listening to the *wake-up* side of the tape an individual is typically refreshed and revitalized. The concise design of the tape includes all representational systems with artfully-vague language patterns. One of the considerations for tape length is usability. A 20-minute tape affords the user greater flexibility in finding time to listen to the tape. The tapes can then become an integral part of a daily break or lunch hour. The tapes are not designed to be listened to while performing other tasks such as driving a car.

Part of the feedback in the weekly sessions should address the client's satisfaction and response to the tapes being used. Find out what the most memorable or enjoyable parts of the tapes are. You can utilize these areas in your live sessions. If there are specific requests you can address them in live sessions or create a specific tape to address the issues.

For example I had a client who had fond memories of being in the mountains. She enjoyed the snow, the cold air, a hot tub and a fireplace. At her request I created a very personalized tape for her. The tape stayed within the parameters of the other tapes. It contained all of the representational systems and embedded commands as well as the specific requests.

Some clients may have favorite tapes or parts of tapes. Other clients may have little or no recollection of what is on the tapes. That's perfect! Either way, whether they can recall the tapes or not. If a person enjoys the tape, that's fine. Sometimes clients report that they were visualizing things before they were even mentioned. Some client's have little or no recollection of the contents of the tapes or sessions at all.

There is a widely held belief that if you have no recollection of a tape or session then it has gone directly into your unconscious mind. This is great, since all learning takes place in the unconscious mind. Our actual goal in *The Body Contouring Programme*™ is to gain acceptance of the unconscious mind.

Progress

Are your clients experiencing the type of results reported in chapter 7 under research results? What physical changes are occurring? What are the client's overall changes? Have they changed any of their goals or desires? How do they feel about these changes? Are they motivated and optimistic? Are you prepared with answers that might be posed to you?

In order to chart the progress being made you may want to have the client keep a daily journal. Have them be very specific if you like. The greater their involvement on a daily basis the greater the unconscious participation becomes. Ask the client to keep track of how many times a day they listened to their tapes. What time of day do they listen to the tapes? Where are they at when they listen to the tapes? What did they eat on any given day? What type of exercise did they perform? What thoughts have they had about their self? What changes have they noticed?

Another important aspect is the continued success and motivation of the client. Point out the progress that the client is making. Reinforce even the slightest change in mental outlook, attitude or physical appearance. As the client acknowledges the changes that they are making they become able to more rapidly and easily create even greater changes. This creates an even more positive and optimistic outlook and disposition.

As the therapist you are the person that your client will trust and rely upon. Are you prepared to answer all of the questions that may come up? You need to do so in a consistently supportive and constructive manner. You must be able to immediately reframe any negativity into a positive accomplishment. As a therapist you need to focus on, and reinforce the positive aspects of the program that the client is experiencing.

Future Pacing

What instructions have you given the client for maintenance? Have you actually used age progression to allow your client to experience all aspects of the changes?

The maintenance program that I developed and utilize consists of extensive positive reinforcement and anchoring. I utilize an almost constant bombardment of unconscious reinforcement. This contains all representational systems. It is designed to utilize aspects and components of everyday life. For example noticing reflections in mirrors, the feel of clothing, ease of movement, positive compliments and conversations both internal and external.

Utilizing age progression allows the therapist to ask the client if there are any additional areas that needed to be addressed at the time of the therapy. Check for congruency in either case. If further changes needed to be made, suggest them. Afterwards future pace once again to check for compliance. Repeat this process until you have a satisfied, congruent, client.

Chapter Eleven

Scripts

Basic Induction

Find yourself now in a comfortable position..

that's right,.. very relaxed...

as you begin by taking in a very deep breath through your nose...

and then let it out through your mouth. That's good.

Now take in another deep breath through your nose...

and this time, as you let it out through your mouth,

make the sound "Haaa...", like in Hawaii.

That's right.

Taking twice as long to exhale as to inhale.

And on your next breath, breathing in deeply through your nose,

hold it briefly,

and as you exhale through your mouth, making the "Haaa..." sound,

let any and all stress leave your body.

That's right.

Totally relaxed, totally free from any concern... totally relaxed. Very good!

And as you continue breathing in this manner,

becoming even more relaxed,

you might now want to take a moment to thank

your unconscious mind

that we are talking to for taking such good care of you for all this time.

That's right, just taking a moment to thank

your unconscious mind for loving you, and caring for you constantly,

every minute, of every hour, of every day ...

and every night...

year after year...

loving you, and caring for you, as it does even now.

Every minute, of every day and every night, just as it does now.

Your unconscious mind loves you,

and will assist you in doing everything,

everything it can do to allow the changes,

to accept, and allow the changes to take place NOW!

That's right! As we address your unconscious mind,

even now the changes are taking place.

As if it could read your mind,

and know the thoughts before you know the thoughts,

you know, the thoughts you know,

that you know about the change

that you know you are making,

as you know you are changing.

You know?!

And now that you know those thoughts...

the ones that you know, you know.

It's time for you to be aware of how those changes are affecting you now...

as you are aware now, of these changes now,

that you are aware of these changes, now,

that you are aware of these changes now that you can see them.

Because even as you can see the changes,

you can feel these changes that you see..

and feel the changes that you feel,

as you see them,

you feel them

as you become aware of how great and complete

these changes are already being made,

 now that you are aware of these changes,

that you have...

are making through these changes right now.

That's right, you have changed, as you are aware now!

... And as you become even more aware of the depth of your breathing,

you realize how really relaxed you are.

Perhaps even more relaxed than the last time you were this relaxed,

even more relaxed now.

And as you are aware of how relaxed you are

you realize that you are so relaxed that you realize

that you no longer realize how relaxed you are,

because you are so relaxed now.

And because you are so relaxed,

beyond being so relaxed so that you can allow all of your other positive creative thoughts to manifest into the physical

into your thoughts,

into your physical body

as the positive results begin to manifest...

to change...

to take form now!

And even as they do you find yourself in even greater control over your life... mentally, emotionally and physically.

Induction - 10 Levels of Relaxation

As you begin to relax now,

find yourself either seated or reclined in a very comfortable position,

taking the time to relax...

and just begin, by closing your eyes...

and beginning to focus...

upon your breath and breathing.

You may choose to breathe in through your nose...

and notice how calm and peaceful that is

and as you exhale...

perhaps choosing to exhale through your mouth, now...

making the Hawai'ian sound of "Haaa".

Breathing in through your nose and feeling relaxed,

and breathing out, feeling even more peaceful, calm and in an even deeper state of relaxation, now...

and notice how effortlessly you continue to breathe in... and out...

going even deeper into a state of relaxation, **NOW**...

that's right,

breathing in calm and tranquil...

breathing out...

even deeper, deeper state of relaxation, NOW

And even as you continue breathing...

I might ask that as you listen to my voice...

as you allow any and all other thoughts,

any other sounds...

anything at all...

to simply allow you to focus more fully and completely upon my voice, NOW.

And perhaps to assist you in doing that,

you might create in your mind's eye

a very large, strong storage room.

And in this storage room you may choose to place any and all thoughts, concerns, or feelings you've had of the day,

taking everything...

all of your experiences from the day,

the total accumulation of your day

and placing them in that very secure room, NOW

And even as you do so...

simply close the very secure door to it, NOW

locking it,

and taking with you the only key,

NOW

Having done so, I would like to ask you if I may speak specifically and directly to your unconscious mind.

The part of your mind that has been taking care of your body so magnificently for so many years.

The part of your mind which has been controlling the breathing

and the blood flow

and the cell formation and regeneration,

and, indeed,

even the transformation of your body...

from one point in life to another.

From one time to another,

from one size and shape to another...

and realizing that through the normal process of replacement, NOW..

your cells are constantly regenerating and realigning.

Allowing your body to constantly be refreshed and replenished

with healthy, new cells.

I would like to acknowledge the part of your, unconscious mind...

in charge of all of those aspects...

for doing such a wonderful job.

I would also like your unconscious mind

to allow your body to totally relax,

and allowing the unconscious mind to remain sharp and alert...

listening to my voice, NOW

And if you would, NOW,

as you prepare to move to the tenth stage of relaxation...

the tenth stage which is the level of transformation...

where you are one with creation

and yourself, NOW

And as we prepare to do so,

you may begin...

by imagining in your mind's eye...

a very brilliant, bright, white light...

beginning to filter into the room.

A light so bright... so intense and so magnificent,

that everything else pales and fades into the light...

just allowing the white light...

so brilliant...

to be all encompassing.

And all you can see is this

magnificent, warm, nurturing white light surrounding you...

feeling it surrounding your body...

warm and nurturing.

Feeling yourself peaceful and tranquil

and nurtured by this white light, NOW

Now you notice how wonderful, calm and tranquil you feel...

as you begin to allow and sense the white light beginning to move right in through the top of your head...

beginning to slowly...

flowing in... relaxing every cell...

every nerve... and every muscle,

as it begins to enter down into the top of your head...

loving, healing and nurturing,

as it flows down your forehead,

the sides of your head,

and the back of your head, now...

slowly flowing down...

relaxing your scalp,

relaxing and rejuvenating your hair,

every little hair follicle...

being surrounded, caressed and nurtured by this white light...

as it continues flowing down

to your eyebrows,

flowing down and relaxing your temples,

allowing every cell...

every nerve...

every muscle...

every minute, little muscle,

to be totally and peacefully relaxed, now...

as the white light begins to flow down the back of your head,

relaxing your ears...

flowing down to your eyelids...

allowing them to become very heavy... now.

Very relaxed...

and you notice that at any time you would choose you could easily open them...

but for now you simply choose to allow them to remain closed,

relaxed and peaceful...

as you enter into the first stage of relaxation,

now.

As you notice the white light flowing down the bridge of your nose,

around the tip of your nose... and around your nostrils..

flowing out across your cheeks...

and your upper lip,

flowing out and relaxing your jaw...

and on down to all your facial muscles...

nurtured, soothing, relaxing every nerve, cell and muscle.

The white light relaxes your lips and your chin,

and you may even sense your mouth falling open...

or your teeth separating...

or even your tongue falling back in your mouth,

and even as you swallow,

you might find yourself even more relaxed...

in this second stage of relaxation,

NOW

And noticing just as you swallow,

the white light does indeed flow down...

down your throat...

soothing, nurturing...

down the back of your neck...

relaxing every part of your neck...

feeling your head and neck firmly, comfortably supported...

feeling yourself nurtured,

supported comfortably and relaxed...

as the white light flows down both of your shoulders...

allowing every muscle to relax...

every cell...

and every nerve.

To become even more relaxed,

in this, the third stage of relaxation.

Even sensing your shoulders falling back

being supported comfortably and peacefully,

as you allow the white light to begin to flow down into your right shoulder

your upper arm,

your right elbow...

your right forearm,

flowing easily and effortlessly down

your right arm...

all the way to your right wrist,

feeling your right arm becoming heavier,

heavier with the white light relaxing all the cells, nerves and muscles...

as the white light flows on down into your right wrist and your right palm,

feeling the white light all the way in the back of your right hand...

moving into your right thumb...

your right index finger...

relaxing every joint along the way,

relaxing the middle finger...

your ring finger...

and your little finger, now

as you sense the white light

soothing...

relaxing...

tranquil...

flowing out the fingertips and back

into the oneness of the white light in the room... in this,

the fourth stage of relaxation...

and even as... you notice that...

you become even more aware of your left shoulder...

and begin to wonder if its heavier than the right...

or if the right, is heavier than the left...

as the white light flows down and relaxes it...now...

perhaps even more than the right side

the left side is relaxed,

as the white light flows down into the left elbow,

relaxing every cell and muscle along the way...

healing and nurturing,

the white light flows down

into the right... left... right.... left... forearm,

and into the left wrist and hand

relaxing and healing your entire body

as the white light flows into the palm and back of your left hand...

into your left thumb...

and into every knuckle and joint...

into the index finger...

the middle finger...

the ring finger...

and the little finger,

of the left hand.

You notice now how

heavy, peaceful, tranquil and relaxed

your left arm is...

and you may not be able to tell if the left or the right arm...

is more relaxed now.

As the white light flows out the fingertips of your left hand,

and into the room...

as you feel the white light, now, in the fifth... stage of relaxation...

begin to slowly flow down your back...

that's right...

just relax,

your shoulder blades... your wing bones...

very soothing white light...

flowing down your back...

caressing your spinal column...

all the way down...

your adrenal glands...

relaxing, healing, soothing and nurturing...

all the way down to your kidneys...

all the way down...

relaxing all the muscles in your back, now.

All cells and all the nerves,

all the micro muscles...

all the way down to the small of your back...

soothing... nurturing...

the healing white light...

flowing down,

in this, the sixth stage of relaxation

As you sense now the white light flowing down your chest,

relaxing your collarbone and your ribs...

and feeling the white light flowing down into your breasts...

allowing them to become heavier...

more relaxed now...

as the healing white light flows...

all around into your heart...

healing, loving and nurturing...

loving the white light through your entire body, now

as this healing white light caresses all of your lungs

entering them; filling them

with healing, balancing loving white light

relaxing, soothing

continuing to move all the way down into your abdomen now

relaxing and loving; healing and nurturing all of your internal organs, now

the white light slowly flowing and healing

moving all the way down to your stomach; your liver; your pancreas; your spleen;

all of your internal organs

healing all the way down to your intestines

as the white light flows down nurturing all of your body

in this seventh stage of relaxation, now

as you feel the white light flowing down into your hips

flowing from your waist down into your hips

flowing all the way down into your pelvis

flowing down into your sexual organs

relaxing, healing, nurturing

flowing on down into your right and your left buttocks

down into your right and your left thigh

healing, nurturing and relaxing

allowing the right or.... is it the left.... to become heavier now

as they both become so relaxed and peaceful

as the white light flows

healing, loving energy

down into your right and your left knee

in this, the eighth stage of relaxation, now

as you feel the white light flowing down your legs

all the way down your shins and into your calves

the white light flows down into your ankles

into your right and your left foot, now

feeling the white light flowing, healing and loving

nurturing your right heal and your left heal

nurturing and loving and healing

relax every cell; every nerve and every muscle of your right foot and your left foot

simultaneously

down the instep and the arch;

the ball of the foot

and all ten toes

simultaneously

as the white light flows

flows on down

into the remainder of the room

in this, the ninth stage of relaxation, now

as you feel the oneness of the light

the oneness of the room

and all the light surrounding and nurturing

as if one with you

and as you take a moment

as I count backwards from five to one

just make a quick, little review of your body

and notice how totally and completely relaxed you are

and should you find any area of tension

just allow it to relax

going over your whole body, now

as I count backwards from five

to four

realizing how totally relaxed and peaceful you are

as you go even deeper into relaxation

from four

to three

calmer

allowing your body to naturally heal itself

free

and yet your mind is so alert

focusing upon my voice

with two

and going all the way down

ten times deeper now

with one

that's right

deeply

into the ninth stage of relaxation, now

and as you prepare to move on

move on down into the tenth level of relaxation

move down to the room

of transformation

and prepare to move down the ten steps

as I count them off

moving comfortably

securely down the steps

to the tenth level of relaxation

and trance formation

going ten times deeper still

with each decreasing number, now

as you move from the tenth step

down onto the ninth

allowing yourself to totally relax

down onto the eighth step

moving slowly

and relaxed

down onto the seventh step

as you continue down to the fifth... or is it the sixth...

that's right...

down onto the sixth step

and you know that you're half way there, now

on the fifth step

where you can now see the dimly lit room at the bottom

as you move down onto the fourth step

and your anticipation becomes even greater

as you're excited as you move down deeper

from the fourth step to the third

and on deeper still

finding yourself ten times deeper than you've ever found yourself before

from the third step onto the second

as you stand there looking at the first step

between you and the landing

your realize that you're almost there

and you can go a hundred times deeper

in relaxation with this next step, now

onto the first step, now

deeper into relaxation

and trance-formation

than you have ever been before

as you move on down onto the landing

having come all the way down

all the way down to the tenth level

the tenth stage of relaxation, now

the stage where all transformation takes place

and now that you've arrived

you know what you came here to do

in this, the tenth stage of relaxation

and so we'll give you the opportunity to allow those changes to take place

because when you are in the tenth level... the tenth stage of relaxation

you know that you're beyond time and space

and that all things are now

and that by simply having the thought you now possess that thought

that all change is now

and that you, the unconscious mind in charge of all change

can accept that change, now

and so whenever you choose to

change now

you can

in this, the tenth stage of relaxation,

now

and I'd like to suggest that should you and I choose to work together again

if that would be appropriate for you

and should l be willing

and agreeable on both parts

that we would allow you to enter into this, the tenth stage of relaxation

instantaneously

since all time is now

and in order for us to do that

I'd like to ask if it would be alright

for me to simply use the word "relax"

or perhaps I can pose the question to you, "Would you like to relax?"

or "Could you relax, now?"

If that would be acceptable to you

that would be acceptable to me

and being acceptable to you is important

so simply give me a sign by perhaps, a nod of the head

and let me know that would be acceptable to you, now

that's right

thank you

very good, then

should you and I choose to work together again

at any time

and you would be agreeable

and I would be agreement

I would simply ask you to relax and

enter into the tenth stage of relaxation

and you may find that would be appropriate for you to do

at any time you choose to listen to any of these tapes

we have made specifically for you

that at the beginning I would simply ask you to relax

at which point you would go into the tenth stage of relaxation

or even deeper

when I simply ask you to relax

and go into the tenth stage of relaxation or even deeper

and knowing that you and I have entered into an agreement on that

I'll leave it with that; leave it with you

and I'll simply ask you to relax and go into the tenth level of relaxation

or perhaps even deeper into that level of trance-formation, now

and with that I would ask you now

to begin to move from the room of trance-formation

and begin to go up the stairway

from the tenth level of relaxation

stepping onto the first step

and up to the second

continuing along up to the third

and to the fourth

moving on to the fifth;

the sixth;

and the seventh step

on up to the eighth step

and the ninth

and back up to the top

and the tenth step and the landing

where you find yourself in the ninth stage of relaxation

aware of your body as you

allow the white light begin to leave

as it comes up through all ten toes and up through your feet

leaving through the top of your head

leaving you relaxed, nurtured and healed

feeling the white light flowing up your legs

healing and flowing up through your knees

moving up through both your right and your left thigh, now

leaving them both relaxed, soothed and comfortable

as the white light flows up through your pelvis; your sexual organs;

and your buttocks; up through your waist and your hips

feeling the white light flowing up

from the eighth to the seventh level

up through your abdomen; your internal organs

leaving them relaxed and healed

moving out through your chest; your lungs and your heart

flowing up through your breasts

leaving them healthy, symmetrical and in perfect health

as the white light flows up your back

up from the small of your back

from your kidneys and adrenal

all the way up the spinal cord and the wing bones

moving on up feeling the white light flowing up through your left hand;

through the fingers; the palm; the back of your hand and wrist

as the white light flows up your forearm, into your elbow and your upper arm

... your left hand now and up through your fingertips;

your palm; the back of your right hand and your wrist;

flowing up through your forearm; your elbow and up to your shoulder

as the white light begins to leave now

up to your shoulders; across your back

and up the back of your neck and throat

as the white light leaves the third and the second stage of relaxation

moving up your face

relaxing your entire jaw and your face

as the white light flows up

through your eyes and your nose

and up through your forehead

as the white light enters back into the room from your body

leaving you relaxed and peaceful as the white light dissipates from the room

bringing you back into the room

recalling our agreement

that at whatever time we would choose to work together again

I would simply ask you to relax

and enter into.... this tenth stage of relaxation or perhaps even deeper

and for now I'm going to ask you to go forward in your day

fully refreshed and revitalized

as though you've had an entire evening's restful sleep

and at which point it is time for your to go to sleep

you do so easily and peacefully

awaking at the appropriate time in the morning

as I count forward now from one to five

at five you will find yourself wide awake, alert and refreshed

not yet

but in just a moment

as I move forward from one to five

you'll find yourself wide awake, alert and refreshed

with complete understanding of all processes which were appropriate for you

to allow you to enter into the tenth stage of trance-formation now

I'll simply ask you to relax

at which point you'll go into that tenth stage of relaxation or

perhaps even deeper now

as we prepare to move forward now

from one to five

at five finding yourself wide awake, alert and refreshed

moving forward now from one to two

and with the simple number two

you become more aware of your body

and as we move from two to three

you find yourself things around you

sensations

perhaps even sounds around the room

as we move from three to four

becoming more refreshed and revitalized

now

taking a very deep breath

breathing comfortably and normally now

very peaceful

as we move from four to five

opening your eyes at any time

finding yourself wide awake, alert and refreshed

with normal movement returning to your body

wide awake, alert and refreshed as if you've had an entire evening's sleep

good job

very good, indeed.

The Private Cove

[Having already done a deep induction.]

.... Find yourself, now,

lying back,

comfortable and warm...

 in your own very secluded,

private,

comfortable cove at the beach.

Lying back,

on a nice.. soft... warm towel,

being gently supported by the warm sand,

contouring beneath your body.

And as you lie back,

feeling the sun above...

beating down on your body...

notice how you feel very, very warm.

Almost as if you're baking in the sun.

You know...

the kind of warm when you just start to glisten or glow,

with the slightest bit of... perhaps perspiration upon your skin.

And yet you are aware of the lightest...

most gentle bit of breeze coming off the ocean,

and cooling you with a temperature that is juuuust right.

And as you lie back feeling the sun upon your face;

upon your breasts;

upon your abdomen;

your thighs; your legs; your arms...

and this heat soaking into you...

this warm, golden, glowing light...

Its almost as if it passes right in through the top of your head...

flowing through your entire body,

filling it all...

filling it all up...

as you become aware of the sounds of the sea;

of the wind blowing...

and the constant pulsing and vibration of the ocean.

As water slides up the sand and across...

and just slips back down into the sea once again.

As you notice how the sound of the sea...

ebbing and flowing...

pulsing constantly back.. and forth...

and down upon the shore...

And as it does...

so you realize your own heart pumps your blood back and forth ...

and up and down through your body.

And just like the sea that carries so many things so far,

and deposits them upon the shore...

your blood does the same thing...

with all of the oxygen and nutrients within your body.

Moving all the nutrients around in your body,

delivering and depositing them in the parts of your body,

 where they are most desired and needed now.

And even as you are aware of this...

and your breathing,

you smell the freshness of the salt air on your body...

feel the dampness of the humidity,

mixing with your own skin.

You realize that your body is mostly made up of water,

and that the 96 elements in the seawater are the same,

as the 96 elements in your blood.

And that in many ways you are one with the sea...

as it pulses,

as it ebbs and it flows...

constant...

constant, to and fro...

ever changing,

and yet...

basically the same.

And just as the sea will move to and from the shore,

removing and depositing sand...

changing the shoreline...

changing the shapes and contours of the shoreline...

you, yourself, begin to shape and change the contours of your own parameters.

Your own shoreline meets the water;

your own body grows cells.

Realizing that not unlike the process of baking in the sun...

as you are now...

baking a cake,

and things begin to rise with the proper ingredients...

 in the proper proportions, now.

And in your own body...

in the proper proportions, now,

you feel a shift in the sand beneath you.

As you begin to move just slightly,

to allow the contours of the sand to align with the contours of your body...

as you feel that warmth;

that firmness around your back...

the small of your back;

your buttocks;

the backs of your thighs, and calves and knees...

feeling the support across your back;

your adrenal;

your kidneys...

the warmth coming up from the earth through the sand;

 supporting your shoulders;

the back of your neck;

the back of your head...

As you feel the sun up above, and the light...

the golden, warm light...

coming down onto your head;

onto your face...

replenishing and rejuvenating the moisture in your skin;

the moisture from the sea;

the moisture from creation...

all about you, now.

Its as though you feel any signs of aging...

wrinkling...

beginning to melt;

beginning to disappear and melt like butter in the sun...

smoothing out...

every so soft and silky...

as a light breeze just begins,

to blow away any wrinkles that may have even tried to form.

And notice that even as it moves across the body,

and keeps it soft, and supple and cool...

finding how silky smooth and soft your skin is.

And aware of the smoothness moving right on down your face;

down your neck;

your throat...

feeling how soft and supple...

and yet,

how elastic the skin is;

how youthful, in fact, it feels, now.

As it connects around your chest;

your collarbone;

and across your breasts...

feeling the sunlight on your breasts, and the warmth created in your chest.

Realizing how your chest raises and lowers with your breath...

as it becomes more rapid and deeper now.

Notice the deeper the breath you take,

the more your chest expands;

the higher the breasts are elevated into the air,

and the higher they become above your body...

the more the breeze... begins to interact with them.

Feel the coolness of the breeze across your breasts;

across your nipples;

contrasting with the heat of the sun...

the glowing, shining wetness;

the moistness of your skin in the sun...

constantly being cooled;

constantly being warmed...

as the process goes...

to eliminate excesses and toxins to your skin...

the breath increases the flow of oxygen into your lungs;

into your bloodstream;

and into your breasts, now.

And even as you breathe...

you feel the blood flow increasing into your breasts...

where all of the blood vessels and veins are expanding now...

not unlike tributaries to a river,

as they begin to swell and overflow with enormous presence of energy

and nutrients now being pumped into your breasts...

allowing them to become fuller, firmer and larger.

And with each inhalation you take, its like pumping up a bicycle tire...

as your breasts become fuller,

firmer....

that's right...

in perfect symmetry... now.

Notice that even as they become even larger and fuller,

now...

they become even more sensual...

and even the presence of the breeze across your nipples is extremely
sensitive and sensual... now.

Be aware of this.

Be also aware that just one cell may split and become two,

and two become four;

four become eight;

eight become sixteen,

which then becomes thirty-two;

becoming sixty-four;

becoming a hundred twenty-eight;

becoming two hundred fifty-six;

and on and on and on and on...

faster and faster;

multiplying...

up to seven million cells a day,

replaced in your body...

now.

And you...

the unconscious mind...

that's right...

you...

the unconscious mind...

are aware of how to increase this even more rapidly...

now.

That is, indeed, your charge;

your concern;

your responsibility...

just as you have maintained the body right along...

and now given direct charge to realign the body;

to change the outward physical representation,

and realize what extremely powerful...

now...

the power of knowledge;

the power of maturity;

the power of your own understanding coupled with the energy and suppleness of youth...

now.

....a stronger; a more powerful; more glorious you....

find that even your energy level increases in every way...

with every beat of your heart...

feeling stronger and stronger...

feeling that pulsing in your breasts;

around your heart;

stronger and stronger;

as the life force in your body is increasing as you vibrate ever closer to that of the light;

to that of the sun...

very good...

very good, in deed.

And as you notice the blood flow increasing in your breasts,

you are also aware of the sensation increasing;

the vibration increasing throughout your entire body,

now.

Realize that all processes have been sped up;

realizing that circulation increases all the way from the tip of your toes to the top of your head...

and all points in between.

Realize that,

almost as though you were squeezing a tube of toothpaste,

you find that as your body firms up...

from your toes on up through your legs;

feeling the firming of your thighs;

your buttocks;

as though you were squeezing everything upwards;

moving upwards into your breasts.

Feel the cells increasing along the way...

becoming healthier and healthier;

Realizing that in only 30 days you have an entirely new, youthful skin now.

Realizing that your normal process of elimination,

repair and replacement,

they are all...

at work...

representation of your body...

of the new,

now.

Knowing this...

you feel your body being smoothed...

warmed...

in the sun.

Be aware of anything that was once interpreted or perceived as an imperfection,

has melted away in the sunlight.

And through the normal process of elimination,

as you are reading your body...

being replaced with the perfect blueprint of health...

with the perfect image of you...

as you know you've created to be,

now.

Only as soon as you are aware of all these changes being aligned,

and your body accepting them,

now,

will you find yourself with the means to sit upright,

looking around this very private beach;

very secure...

in complete control you move upright,

onto your feet....

feeling all of that warmth of the sand...

almost hot ...

to the touch...

You almost prance down to the water,

and you feel the weight of your breasts having increased...

the fullness in the way they move with your body.

Movement...

the weight of your breasts upon your chest...

the way the skin pulls ever so slightly up on your shoulders and beneath your arms and the sides....

the tautness from your breasts going down into your ribs to your solar plexus...

the excitement and sensuality of your nipples in the breeze...

as you sense the cool, wet, moist sand beneath your feet...

as you get closer to the water...

closer to the edge of the sea.

Begin to slowly enter ...

feeling the water flowing up around your ankles...

cooling and soothing...

yet, just a refreshing warm temperature...

that's perfect now...

Feeling it swirling around your feet and up your legs...

supporting and cleansing your calves and your shins...

and notice how soothing it is as it gets up to your knees

as the movement of the ocean is massaging all of the joints...

and your body relaxes.

Sense the support of your knees as the water moves up your thighs...

and notice the tautness of your thighs...

notice how firm they've become...

notice the tonicity of your skin...

so soft and supple...

now, as you discharge all of the excess into the sea.

You feel your genitals beginning to be cooled by the water as the water moves up to your buttocks and over your abdomen and waist...

feeling the coolness swirling and churning around you...

the tingling sensation,

as you begin...

slowly...

to move up to your breasts...

into the sea,

feeling the sand between your toes...

feeling the cleansing action...

the abrasive nature of the sand,

and the feel of the sand...

suspended in the water...

flowing all about you...

helping your body to exfoliate the excesses...

allowing the pulsing and movement of the sea to cleanse and purify you now.

Feel your breasts beginning to enter into the sea,

and feel the buoyancy that takes place with your perfectly proportioned breasts, now.

And the titillating sensation as your nipples,

with the coolness of the water...

feel sensation,

now.

As the weight is released from your chest...

as your breasts are floating now in the water,

as you, yourself, are floating in the water...

being nurtured in this pulsing, flowing, endless source of power...

not unlike being supported in the womb,

with all nutrients you need within the seawater...

cleansing, cooling, refreshing, embracing you in the water...

Experiencing the ocean all around you...

supporting you,

cleansing you,

vibrating with you...

as you are one with the sea,

now.

Once again,

just as this power of the sea...

the force moves...

the shifting sand like the shifting cells within your body,

realign them on the shoreline...

removing them,

and replacing them...

constantly,

as does your unconscious mind,

now.

Realign the shapes;

the patterns;

the outward representation of your physical body...

just as the shoreline upon the beach changes.

as does that of your body,

now.

Where are those changes having taken...

place your head and your face to the water once...

feeling the water streaming down through your hair;

giving it strength...

health...

vitality

feeling the water....

cleansing across your face...

giving it a new youthful appearance and glow.

As you find yourself, now...

comfortable,

confident and relaxed.

Full of energy as you move towards the beach...

begin to emerge from the water,

and as you do so,

you feel the water streaming down your neck onto your shoulders...

down your back and your buttocks...

Feel the water rolling down your chest;

your breasts and around your breasts.

And as you stand there,

looking down toward your feet,

you notice the parts of your body that are obscured from vision because of the largeness of your breasts now...

the fullness and the increase...

the absolutely perfect,

perfect balance...

perfect size;

perfect shape;

and the perfect proportions of your body,

now...

as the water streams down your abdomen;

your thighs....

the sunlight begins to bake you dry once again,

as you move,

and in the slight breeze across the shoreline...

seeing your own reflection in the water ...

of perfection...

and looking and seeing your own shadow and silhouette upon the sea;

upon the shore;

shadow upon the beach,

as you turn...

playfully...

from side to side...

and see the silhouette change...

representing your own change upon the sand...

the shifting sand that shifts as easily as the cells of your body...

now...

to conform to your perfect figure,

now.

And feeling refreshed and revitalized,

now,

you move to your towel...

drying yourself...

and finding yourself absolutely free...

free and refreshed...

you perhaps reach into your bag,

spray or rub on a bit of lotion...

scintillating your skin,

and notice that as you rub your own hand across your body...

you feel the energy present,

you feel the stimulation for growth and for change...

particularly as you run your hand across the areas of change,

as you feel your breasts in the palms of your hands...

and the tips of your fingers...

you feel the tingling sensation both in your breasts...

and in your hands...

and you feel the connectedness within your body...

as your body...

lovingly...

transforming now.

And even as you are being aware of this,

you rub lotion or spray down upon your body...

across your abdomen...

over your hips...

your buttocks....

your thighs and legs...

down your arms...

indeed,

your hands and feet...

fully anointed with this wonderful...

wonderful...

lotion.

Locking in the changes now,

and allowing more changes to occur.

Feeling light and playful and fully energized,

you slip into a light,

little sundress...

and you are aware that even the fabric...

on your body stimulates growth and sensuality...

and as you move,

and feel the fabric upon your body...

the tingling continues and increases...

being a sign that,

indeed,

change is occurring,

now.

Every movement you make...

every time the fabric touches any part of your body,

you become even more keenly aware of it,

now.

Each time you are aware of it,

the change is deepened on even deeper levels now...

allowing all changes...

mental,

emotional and physical...

to take place...

in conjunction now for the highest good...

now.

As you gather up your belongings,

and begin to walk along the edge of the sea once again...

playfully,

lightly...

in your own magnificence...

moving along...

feeling your oneness with the sun...

your oneness with the sea....

oneness with the sand

moving towards the point ahead,

around which you return to the public beach.

And as you come around that point,

notice people becoming aware of your presence.

And knowing that you are the goddess...

the perfection...

the absolute,

magnificent you...

you and you alone,

are given access to that private bay around the point...

a place that you may return at any time...

but is yours and yours alone...

your place of transformation....

now.

And as you move up the beach towards the parking lot,

you can feel,

sense,

and notice the admiring approving glances...

see others perceptions of you...

almost an enviousness towards you,

a lovingness towards you...

you may even hear polite comments...

soft conversation between others in reference to you,

and how accepted they are...

and desirous they are to be with you,

or be like you...

now.

Feeling all of this...

sharing all of this...

knowing all of this...

moving through the parking lot...

moving on to where you need to go,

now....

References

Brown, B.B. *"New Mind, New Body"*, New York: Harper and Rowe, 1974.

Brown, W.E. *Stimulation of Breast Growth by Hypnosis, Journal of Sex Research*, 1974, 10:316-326.

Bullard, Barbara; Carroll, Kat, *Communicating From The Inside Out*, Kendall/Hunt Publishing Company, 1993.

Capra, Fritjof, *The Tao of Physics*, 3rd edition, updated, Shambala Publications, Inc, Boston, Massachusetts, 1991.

_____ , *The Turning Point, Siene, Society and the Rising Culture*, Bantam Books, New York 1982.

Chopra, Deepak, *Ageless Body, Timeless Mind*, Harmony Books, New York, 1993.

_____ , *Quantam Healing, Exploring the Frontiers of Mind/Body Medicine*, Bantam Books, New York, 1989.

Davies, Paul, *God and the New Physics*, Simon and Schuster, New York, 1983.

Dyer, Wayne, W., *Your Erroneous Zones*, HarperCollins, New York, 1976.

Ferris, Timothy, *The World Treasury of Physics, Astronomy and Mathematics*, Little, Brown & CO., 1991.

James, E. Tad; Woodsmall, Wyatt, *Time Line Therapy and the Basis of Personality*, Meta Publications, Cupertino, CA, 1988.

Maltz, Max well, *Psycho-Cybernetics*, Prentice-Hall, Inc.,1960.

Mutke, P. H. C., Research paper on the subject of *Mental Techniques for Breast Development*, Presented to the department of Neuropsychiatry, University of California, Los Angeles, 2/28/71.

Peat, F. David, *The Philosopher's Stone*, Bantam, New York, 1991.

Pelletier, Kenneth R.; Herzing, Denise L.,*Psychoneuroimmunology: Toward a Mind-Body Model*, taken from: *Eastern & Western Approaches to Healing & Ancient Wisdom & Modern Knowledge*, Sheikh & Sheikh, Eds., John Wiley & Sons, 1989.

Rossi, Ernest L., *The Psychobiology of Mind-Body Healing*, W. W. Norton & Co., Inc; New York, 1988.

Staib, A.R. & Logan, D.R. *Hypnotic Stimulation of Breast Growth*, *American Journal of Clinical Hypnotherapy*, 19:201 1977.

Talbot, Michael, *The Holographic Universe*, HarperCollins, New York, 1991.

Wilben, Ken, *The Revolution of Consciousness*, taken from; *Beyond Health & Normality*, R. Walsh & D. Shapiro, Eds., New York: Van Nostrand, 1983.

Willard, R. D., *Breast Enlargement Trough Visual Imagery and Hypnosis, American Journal of Clinical Hypnosis*, 19:195,1977.

Williams, J.E., *Stimulation of Breast Growth by Hypnosis, Journal of Sex Researc*,10:316, 1974.

Wilson, D.L., *Natural Bust Enlargement With Total Mind Power*, Mind Power Institute; Larkspur, California, 1979.

Publisher's Related Books

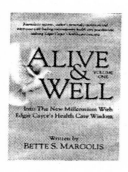

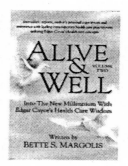

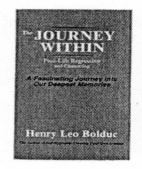

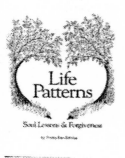

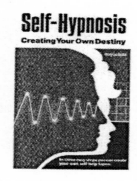

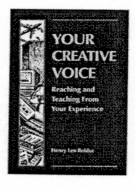

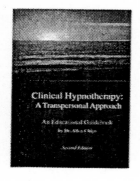

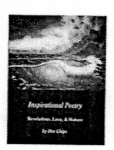

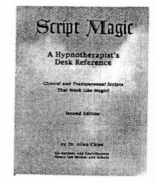

To order direct, contact the publisher:
www.TranspersonalPublishing.com

Additional copies of this book be purchased by contacting Pau Publications at the address below.

Also available is *The Body Contouring Programme*™ Audio Tape Series. This series consists of six twenty-minute cassette tape inductions. These inductions have been developed to provide maximum flexibility and benefit for the listener. They have been clinically proven to assist in accelerating the physical change process. The voice tracks are mixed over a background music that has been clinically developed and proven to provide a sequential relaxing, deepening and opening of the endocrine or chakra systems. The audio tape series is designed to be used independently or in conjunction with the book You're Sharp Enough To Be Your Own Surgeon: The Body Contouring Programme™.

You're Sharp Enough To Be Your Own Surgeon $14.95*

The Body Contouring Programme™ audio tape series $69.95*

Volume discounts are available.

For information on *The Body Contouring Programme*™ seminar or becoming a *Body Contouring Programme*™ Practitioner, information on NLP, Time Line Therapy™, Huna, other trainings and seminars, or to order products please contact us or visit our website at:

About Communication..., Ltd.

888.372.5275 / www.amindfield.com

* prices subject to change

Printed in the United States
40364LVS00006B/125

9 781929 661169